Everyone knows someone who is childle[ss] ... a rare opportunity to get a glimpse of h[ow] ... say and what not to say. For those who s[uffer] ... infertility and its implications, it shows h[ow] ... godly and how, in a way that is neither glib nor trite, to replace self-pity with well-founded trust in a good God.
Ann Benton, pastor's wife, speaker and author

The frankness, the style and the inclusion of male testimonies are all very helpful. I like it!
Andrew Fergusson, Christian Medical Fellowship

It means so much to read Christian thinking on this topic. The authors tackle the complexities of infertility in a way that I found both supportive and challenging. I hope this helps fellow Christians talk more openly, and in a more informed and compassionate way. I wish this had been available to my husband and me earlier in our journey.
Becca O'Brien, adoptive mother

Honest, thoughtful, practical, relevant, and biblical. Written out of painful first-hand experience and imbued with practical Christian wisdom. I highly recommend this sensitive and informative book on such an important but rarely discussed problem. It should be essential reading for couples facing the silent pain of infertility and for pastors, Christian counsellors and all those who seek to help and support.
John Wyatt, Professor of Ethics and Perinatology at University College London and author

Eleanor Margesson & Sue McGowan

Just the two of us?

Help and strength
in the struggle to conceive

ivp

INTER-VARSITY PRESS
Norton Street, Nottingham NG7 3HR, England
Email: ivp@ivpbooks.com
Website: www.ivpbooks.com

First published 2010

British Library Cataloguing in Publication Data
A catalogue record for this book is available from the British Library.

ISBN: 978-1-84474-475-6

Typeset in Great Britain by CRB Associates, Potterhanworth, Lincolnshire
Printed in Great Britain by Ashford Colour Press Ltd, Gosport, Hampshire

*Inter-Varsity Press publishes Christian books that are true to the Bible and that
communicate the gospel, develop discipleship and strengthen the church for its
mission in the world.*

*Inter-Varsity Press is closely linked with the Universities and Colleges Christian
Fellowship, a student movement connecting Christian Unions in universities and
colleges throughout Great Britain, and a member movement of the International
Fellowship of Evangelical Students. Website: www.uccf.org.uk*

Contents

Section 4: The long unknown

Foreword

Ever since I (Rachel) can remember, I have wanted to be a mum, so when Jason and I found that conceiving our own children was going to be nigh impossible, we were devastated.

For a long time we didn't like to think too much about it. It was almost as if in looking too far into our childlessness we would see a future we had never pictured for ourselves – a picture we didn't like. I began to feel that if I started down the path of facing my infertility, I would literally end up in my own womb: untouchable and lost.

Childlessness (of any form) can be deeply painful. And no matter how loving close friends and family are, it is still a profoundly isolating reality. It's hard to find words to talk about it, because it isn't just something you are *going through* – it's a *new identity* in which you need to find yourself, your spouse and God.

This book is written by two women who have found the words to talk about the issue of childlessness, and in reading it we have been comforted and encouraged that we are not alone in waiting for our family.

It takes a very brave couple or individual to look into their childlessness. Eleanor and Sue know what they are asking of us because they have both walked this path, and they are still travelling it. So, in reading this book, you will really feel that you are in the hands of good women who understand what you are facing on a very profound level. They bring their skills, patience, understanding and sensitivity to this issue, which makes them the right companions for everyone travelling the long, hard road of childlessness.

If you are struggling with infertility, then the prospect of reading a book like this might feel like opening a floodgate that you don't know if you are prepared for.

It's understandable to be cautious, but I would gently want to suggest that when you are ready this will be a wonderful book to help you in your struggle. Eleanor and Sue are real, honest, compassionate and wise. They don't tempt you with platitudes or neat solutions. Instead, they invite you to explore God's promise to do you good, even in this.

We hope that as you read this book you will experience the strength that comes in knowing that you are not alone, and that your childlessness doesn't need to have the final word in your life and family; that in the middle of facing all the things that you can't do or have, you *can* begin to embrace all that your heart hopes for.

May this book help you to grieve, to face your new reality, to find hope and to seek out the path to deep peace and wholeness that only God can provide.

And above all, may you know he is walking it with you.

Shalom.

Jason and Rachel Gardner

Meet the authors

This book started when we were asked by a friend to work together on running a seminar on 'Childlessness' at the 2008 London and Northern Women's Conventions. Our aim then was to provide support and teaching for those facing the stresses of infertility: people who were largely on their own with minimum support. We wanted them to know that they weren't alone in their struggle and to try to give them a biblical foundation with direct relevance to their situation which would help them to strengthen their relationship with God. After the conventions, we were approached by IVP and asked to expand our material into the format of a book.

We were keen to do this because we realized that there were many women at the convention (not to mention all the men!) who were facing childlessness but who weren't present at the seminar. It took a lot of courage for many to sign up and come along, particularly when they had not even discussed the issue with friends who were with them at the convention. We felt that a book would make it easier for people to access support, information and teaching. We also thought of many more areas that we should have covered in the first place, which could be explored further in a book.

There are many books on the topics of infertility, miscarriage, late-term and post-natal death. Most of them are profound, moving and well written, often by folk who have experienced more tragic and testing times than we can even imagine. They do great work in drawing alongside men and women as they experience tragedies in their lives, and in sensitively expressing the myriad emotions that run throughout a lifetime of memories and ongoing grief.

So why do we feel the need to add another book to those that already exist? We have found that what is often left out is a comprehensive look at the biblical material that will help to make some sense of infertility in the context of God's whole plan of salvation. Both of us have benefited from good Bible teaching on the issue of suffering, which we have found particularly useful in understanding the reality of God's goodness to us in the midst of heartache. We have learnt that we are not immune from problems, and that we grow as Christians because of them. Most importantly, no matter how awful and difficult it seems, God is in control of what is happening to us, even if we most definitely are not.

We also wanted to write a book that men would be prepared to read, because it is obviously not just women who struggle with this pain. We have decided to include a stand-alone chapter on men, co-written with men, so that they can articulate male-specific concerns and issues. But we hope that it is clear from the outset that every single chapter is written with both male and female readers in mind. We want this to be a book that couples can read and discuss together, without isolating either partner.

We realize that not everyone facing childlessness will want to read this book. We understand that everybody's experience of childlessness is different. Some people will want to rush around, reading everything that there is on the subject. Others will feel utterly paralysed by the idea and simply want to push it to the furthest recesses of their minds. Many will just want to get on with their lives, trusting that God has their future under control. Some will have chosen not to have children. This book does not aim to address their situation.

Our own experiences and situations have been similar in many ways, with different outcomes:

Eleanor and Nick

We had been married for four years before we decided that we wanted to begin a family. A year later when nothing had happened, we had investigative tests and the verdict of 'unexplained infertility' was returned. After three cycles of failed treatment, we decided to sit back for a few months before taking any further steps. About six months later we went forward for adoption, a decision made largely because of the fact that Nick was himself adopted. Fifteen months later, and five years after we had wanted to start having children, a nine-month-old baby boy was placed with us for adoption. About a year later, I gave birth to our daughter.

Sue and Steve

We've been married for seventeen years. About three years into our marriage we tried to have children. After being unable to conceive naturally, we both went for tests and the diagnosis given was 'unexplained infertility'. We went through a few cycles of treatment which were unsuccessful. We decided not to undergo any more fertility treatment after that. We vaguely thought about adoption, but didn't pursue it, not because of any beliefs against adoption, just because neither of us really wanted to. Since then we haven't been able to conceive and haven't looked at any other treatment options.

The structure of this book is set out according to groupings of questions that childless people often have. They reflect the ways in which questions, concerns and difficulties may develop along the way, particularly as couples reach into the future and consider a life without ever having children. However, there is much that we feel is relevant for every step of the way, and we have tried to make the distinction between these sections and other sections when we are speaking just to one particular stage of the 'journey'. We have tried to take into account a broad picture of infertility, recognizing that infertility, miscarriages, late-term deaths, stillbirths and secondary infertility bring both shared and individual responses from men and women.

We have thought a great deal about how we should treat the whole controversial area of reproductive technologies. We know from experience that it is unnerving to find yourself in a meeting or on the phone with a brisk medical professional or a hassled social worker, and realizing that their expectations about how we are about to proceed are different from our own. We need to prepare ourselves to answer their questions without compromising our Christian beliefs. So, in the chapters considering natural and assisted conception and adoption, we are concerned to guide couples to ask the right questions that will help them to make informed choices, rather than stating what those choices should be. We have gone into a little more detail regarding adoption, because the information available sometimes makes people feel as though believers may be viewed negatively by social services. We have tried to demonstrate how, as committed Christians, you have much in your favour that will recommend you to social workers, rather than penalize you.

We expect that there will be some readers who are not facing childlessness for themselves. They may have friends or family members who are currently struggling with childlessness and want to find out more to enable them to get a better idea of what it is really like. We have not addressed these concerned parties directly, but hope that they will be able to glean enough to work out how they can best support others facing childlessness.

We are very grateful indeed to all those who have shared their stories and personal lives with us. We have tried to include examples from a broad range of situations of infertility to reflect the complexity of the condition. We have taken the decision to leave out any reference as to whether or not the couple ended up having children, unless their story talks about them in the context of adoption or secondary infertility. Our concern is to reflect the struggles that exist in people's lives at the moment, and we are keen that your hope will be based on what God has already done for you, rather than what he has done in the lives of others. Obviously the names are pseudonyms, but you know who you are! Thank you so much.

We want to stress that the purpose of this book is not primarily to give you the hope that you will have a baby. Nor do we want only to offer the hope of bearing the pain of infertility more manageably. Even through the inevitably hopeful tones of the section entitled 'How can the professionals help?', the ultimate hope that we long to share is that God has a rich purpose for our sufferings. So our hearts' desire is that this book above all restores your hope in a sovereign God who orders everything for good.

There are no neat solutions to infertility. No book can ever provide you with a definitive end to what you are facing. Our prayer is that as you struggle with these issues you will be able to agree with this verse: 'And we know that in all things God works for the good of those who love him, who have been called according to his purpose' (Romans 8:28).

Eleanor Margesson and Sue McGowan
January 2010

For Nick, Steve and all those
who have told us their stories

1 Introduction

Tom

We have been 'trying' for a baby for a couple of years now. We have worked out schedules and timetables to perform by. It isn't very romantic! Sometimes Rachel's period is delayed and our hopes go up, only to be dashed a couple of days later . . . so we go back to the schedule again. Everyone keeps saying 'Just relax, it will happen naturally', 'Just take it easy', 'Don't get tense – that's the last thing you should do'. We are often regaled with stories of friends of friends who had children long after they had given up hope. Of course people are well meaning, but their advice rings hollow and the stories get increasingly tiresome. We know other couples in a similar situation and draw comfort from them – until they then get pregnant!

A lonely reality

If you have been waiting a little longer than you expected to have a baby, you are not alone. Even though there are people like you and people like Tom and Rachel all around us, the situations that you face daily may make you feel extremely lonely. Right now in our churches and wider communities there are lots of people who are battling with childlessness in many different ways.

Infertility is not a new phenomenon. Down the ages there have always been couples who have found out the hard way that they could not have children. Throughout history, the experience has sent men and women flying off on exactly the same emotional roller coaster as it does today. No culture or civilization has ever been free of it. When you're going through it, you may feel like you're completely on your own and that no-one else understands, but it is a road that has been trodden by many.

The book of Genesis tells us about Rachel, who was the second wife of Jacob and desperate to have a child. Years and years of frustration went by without seeing any children, until at last she became pregnant. At the birth, she cried out, 'God has taken away my disgrace' (Genesis 30:23). If Rachel felt that being childless was a disgrace, she was showing a way of thinking that was deeply rooted in her culture, and her culture isn't the only one that has treated women harshly when they could not provide their husbands with children.

Astonishingly, some ancient cultures put terrible laws into place that allowed men to abandon or even kill women who could not have children. We can also find out about women who were relied on to have children to continue important family lines for political reasons, such as Queen Mary I of England. She never managed to conceive, but the pressure to produce an heir was so great that she had two phantom pregnancies. A service was even held in Westminster Abbey during one of them to give thanks for her 'unborn child'. When these 'pregnancies' turned out to be fake, it was a huge embarrassment. Her husband, Philip of Spain, was so ashamed that he abandoned her to go and fight wars instead.

So there is nothing new about the problem of infertility, but today's medical progress means that we understand a great deal more about it than we used to.

Who is affected by infertility today?

About one in seven couples faces a problem linked to infertility.[1] If the woman is under thirty-five, a couple is termed as 'infertile' if they have not been able to conceive following a year of unprotected sex. About eighty-five out of 100 couples who have regular sex without contraceptives (that means about three or four times a week) will conceive within a year. After two years about ninety-two out of those 100 couples will have conceived. So if you are in the first couple of years of trying unsuccessfully for a baby, you may well get pregnant in the near future. Having said that, it is also the case that there are still eight out of 100 couples who won't have babies in that time.

Newspapers can be really unkind. Some headlines suggest that women who can't have children are the victims of their own bad choices in life, that it is basically their own fault: 'Career women empty nation's sperm banks!' 'Did I wait too long to get pregnant?' 'Government seeks age limit for reproductive treatments'. They accuse women who are 'suddenly' unable to conceive of wanting to 'have their cake and eat it'. The desire to have children at forty becomes less acceptable than it is at thirty, even though one in five children is born to a mother over thirty-five! It seems really harsh, doesn't it, particularly when men are praised for being able to father babies in their old age.

What causes infertility?

There are many different physical reasons why a couple may not be able to conceive or to carry a baby to full term. There may be one stand-alone reason that prevents you from having a baby, but more often there is a combination of factors, some hidden and impossible to diagnose, some blindingly obvious.

The 'simple' action of a sperm meeting an egg and making a baby turns out to be a major obstacle course of potential problems! The processes mentioned below are only the basic starting points for understanding the problems that can arise at different stages of the journey to pregnancy.

The journey of sperm and egg	Some of the basic problems that can cause infertility
Journey of the sperm	*Problems associated with sperm*
Sperm	Insufficient or absent sperm in testicle
	Undescended testicle
	Poor motility of sperm
	Poor quality of seminal fluid
Sperm ejaculated into urethra	Penetration difficulties
	Erectile dysfunction
	Insufficient depth of penetration
	Vaginal abnormality / scarring / vaginismus
Sperm travels through cervix	Cervical mucus too thick / antibodies kill sperm
	Cervical infection / scar tissue creates block

Journey of the egg	Problems associated with the egg
Egg	Too old Immature Endocrine disturbance (hormonal irregularities may cause the egg to be dysfunctional)
Egg leaves ovary follicle	Absent ovaries Polycystic ovaries Irregular or no ovulation Imbalances of the hormones that initiate and control ovulation Early menopause
Egg travels through Fallopian tube	Fallopian tubes blocked with mucus/twisted/filled with scar tissue from infection preventing passage of egg

Sperm and egg meet	Problems associated with fertilization and implantation
Sperm and egg meet, egg is fertilized, resulting embryo implants in wall of uterus and establishes umbilical cord	Eggs do not fertilize Embryos develop abnormally and die Embryos implant in Fallopian tube – ectopic pregnancy Uterus cannot support implantation – fibroids/endometriosis/womb lining inadequate Hormone imbalances Malfunctioning cervix endangers pregnancy Absent uterus

This is not an exhaustive list but it demonstrates how many different diagnoses are covered by this blanket term of 'infertility'. It is no wonder that the emotional responses to our situation are going to be so varied. Some will know precisely why they cannot conceive. Others will never know. For some the prospects of a natural pregnancy are hopeful and positive, while for others there is a firmly closed door.

Infertility is not always easy to understand

It is not always the stereotypical couple in their mid-thirties who experience the grief of infertility. Single men and women feel it too. Single women don't need to be told that their biological clock is ticking! Most of them would love to be married and have children as soon as possible. They are often forgotten in the infertility picture, even though they may be getting near the age when they will be too old to conceive. It's a double crisis for them. They have to try to deal with the implications of life without children as well as life without a husband.

Other medical problems can also have an impact on infertility. Lots of people have been told that at some point in their lives a disease, a condition or a disability may affect their chances of conceiving in later life. Doctors may even advise them that it wouldn't be a good idea to get pregnant at all. Some people know about serious genetic conditions running in their family that their children could possibly inherit.

Other people affected by the pain and pressures related to having children are those who have conceived but then suffered miscarriage. Then there are those who have given birth to one child, but then find it impossible to have another. This is known as 'secondary infertility' and it is hardly ever talked about.

Hope

*Doctors were very keen to point out we should be careful about
contraception. Now that my body had 'worked out what to do',
number two might come along before we were even ready. Those
words have never left me, and their arrogance and falsehood
still riles and torments me. And so began a downward spiral of
misery that I have not yet fully escaped. My son is now almost
seven.*

Attitudes towards infertility in other cultures

If you ever find yourself in a fertility clinic waiting room, you
will probably see people from religious or cultural back-
grounds whose childlessness brings an outspoken shame on
to the wider family. There are those whose traditions and
heritage depend deeply on having an heir, passing on the
family name and having children to look after them in old age.
Yet couples within these communities are affected by the same
physical factors as the rest of us.

Rashma

*I am a second-generation Bangladeshi woman raised in England.
I married a man who had come straight from Bangladesh. I
was unable to have a child and he left me. I remarried. Again,
I was unable to produce a child and the finger was pointed at me.
Again I was deserted. A third time I married, and this time I went
on to have my six children. Yet in my community and amongst my
family, it was seen to be my fault that I was unable to have children
with those first two men. Who knows why it was? Sometimes it's
not simple – maybe it's the chemistry between two people that
stops it working. How did I feel? Oh, we don't do emotions. We
don't do depression. No-one thinks about what it might feel like
for you.*

Consider also the culture in Malaysia where it is considered very important to have a biological child of your own.

> **Ling**
> *We have been married for three years and everyone is asking us when we are going to have kids. We've found through tests that because of irregular ovulation and low sperm count it is unlikely, although not impossible, that we will conceive naturally. Once we've spent some time monitoring ovulation and trying naturally then we'll consider adoption. This was a shock to many of our Malaysian friends, because strong family ties are so important. We were shocked to find how even the church in Malaysia is entrenched in a culture that says that you have to have your own bloodline.*

Why does infertility cause so much pain?

As you have got to know about other couples who cannot have children, you may have been surprised to hear how they are able to accept their situation and to bear it, even welcoming the opportunities that life offers them without children. You may have felt the pressure to be more like them, or perhaps even inadequate, because for you it hurts so much. If this is how you feel, be reassured! Most people struggle on some level with the prospect that they might never have children.

Infertility can have a traumatic effect on our emotional well-being. It can be such a raw and painful subject.

Taken by surprise

Like most forms of suffering in life, we simply don't expect that it will ever happen to us. We have grown up following the patterns of our parents and wider family and friends, which will inevitably include being part of a family and seeing other families grow. We form ideas about what we want our own family to look like, how many children we want, what we will call them, how we will bring them up. As we grow older, we see our friends, brothers, sisters and cousins all having children. We anticipate that one day we will experience the same thing, unless we have always known of a problem that is going to make it tricky. If we assume that everything is normal, we may get to the right point in life when we feel ready. We come off the contraceptives. Then nothing. We begin to realize that all we had assumed and prepared for may actually be a little longer coming than we had anticipated. Perhaps even the thought sets in, with horror, that we may not have any children at all. Why isn't this happening for me when it is happening so easily for everybody else?

Catherine

When Luke finally agreed that we were ready for parenthood, two years into our married life, things didn't go quite as we had anticipated. The months passed by, the pregnancy tests weren't needed, the pressures on our relationship and, in particular, our sex life, spiralled. All this time, friends around us were announcing the birth of children. When a very close friend of mine and my sister-in-law, who had both had trouble conceiving and in whom I confided, both then fell pregnant, I felt a strange sense of betrayal. Of course I was delighted for them all, but I do remember well the pain that accompanied sharing in their delight.

The regular reminder

When you are waiting a long time to fall pregnant, your period can become your worst enemy. I (Eleanor) remember feeling each month that it was mocking me, telling me that all those hopes I had had for the last three weeks were empty. I had regularly fantasized that this or that twinge was proof of pregnancy, but all the time the opposite was true. It often struck me that the side effects of a period – cramps, low moods and irritability – increased the intensity of the shock that I wasn't pregnant. It made it harder to cope with and made me more miserable to live with. I often found that my anger sometimes led to cleaning the house from top to bottom – perhaps because it was something that I had control over. I would be weepy and morose, and I would need to reassure Nick that I wasn't angry with him. It seemed unfair that the days around the onset of a period were the days when I lacked emotional and physical energy, yet those were the times when I needed it the most.

I wonder if you, like many others trying for a baby, find yourself focusing on trying different things each month to get pregnant. You may have put loads of money, time, effort, sacrifice, embarrassment and determination into a given month's effort. When the period arrives, all of that investment is swept away, quite literally, down the pan. When this cycle is repeated time and time again, you can both feel deeply let down, perhaps by one another, perhaps by yourself, or perhaps by God. Maybe it would have been different if I hadn't been so energetic on the running machine. Maybe I would be pregnant if I wasn't working so hard. Maybe we had sex on the wrong day. Maybe my shower was too hot. It can either trigger more obsessions or lead to an irresolvable sadness with no hope on the horizon.

Amy is in the position where she doesn't even know how long her cycle will be each month. At least I knew that mine was about twenty-six days. I had a relatively short time to wait to find out if I was pregnant. She sometimes finds herself waiting for three months!

Amy

*Thirty-three . . . thirty-four . . . thirty-five . . . when it gets to forty
days I'll do a pregnancy test – this time it might be different. After all
I did feel a bit off earlier . . . could it be the start of morning sickness?
Day forty – I'm not pregnant according to the test. Maybe it's wrong?
It does say it is only 99% accurate . . . I could be the 100th! I'll just
try another test – it still says negative. Maybe I would have been late
anyway, so it could be too early to do the test. I'll try again at day fifty.
Day fifty – negative. Day sixty – negative. My body is playing tricks on
me again. It's hard to know whether I'm late or not, possibly pregnant
or not, as my cycle can be anything from thirty to ninety days.*

There are many women who, like Amy, have to wait longer
than a month. No wonder that women get obsessed by their
childlessness and preoccupied by pregnancy, when each day
holds so much potential for hope or for despair. No wonder
that when people advise you to 'Relax – it will just happen
when you least expect it', you feel like throttling them!

Is this my fault?

Trevor

*Guilt is huge because your thoughts can quickly follow down
the line of, 'What have I done in my past that has caused this?
Am I being judged?' I felt like Stacey would have been better off
marrying someone else, because it was me that had the problem.*

If the doctors find that there is something wrong with one of
you and not the other, it can become very difficult. Seeing
the one that you love crippled with desire for the one thing
that you are not able to give can lead to despair and difficulty
in communication. A study has shown that marriages are
under more stress if the problem lies with the man.[2] One

husband confided to his friend that he might as well be castrated because he could not give his wife what she most wanted. Guilt can tear people apart within themselves, as well as tearing them from one another.

Phil
I got so angry that I found myself carrying on shouting at my wife, even while she was crying. It shocked me that it could ever have got this bad.

If we are feeling angry, then we may long to blame each other. We certainly often take our anger out on each other. This is easier to do if one or other of the couple is feeling less bothered about the lack of children. It can be even trickier if the fertility problem has potentially been caused by lifestyle choices made in the past: an infection resulting from an STD (sexually transmitted disease); a previous unwanted pregnancy that ended in a termination; your body may have gone through the rigours of developmental issues resulting from an eating disorder. The temptation is to find a solid reason for your predicament, but the reality is that a clear reason may never be known. Childlessness can fill the whole horizon with its demand on our emotions, but there are other demands on us, such as our marriage, which we need to be careful not to neglect.

We also have emotional demands made on us by our friends, relatives and churches. We belong to various communities who need us to be part of them. You may struggle with this and, like Elspeth and Kath, find yourself wanting to avoid some kinds of social occasions:

Elspeth
We missed the wedding of an old friend recently because we had just found out the result of a failed cycle of treatment. We couldn't bear

the thought of so many people wanting to catch up with us and asking us how we were and what was going on in our lives. There would be no easy way of telling them about our predicament, and no escaping the sadness that we felt as we tried to avoid that line of questioning.

Kath

Being married to a church minister, I have certain duties. On a Sunday, it is expected that I will be there welcoming visitors and smiling at all I meet. This is not something I begrudge, and I find it a joy. That is, until I have a wobbly day and hear the news of another pregnancy, or a pregnancy of someone who got married last year, or see families with five children and wonder why God has chosen to give those parents so many, or when someone is stressed with their children for misbehaving and says, 'You must be glad you don't have kids when they start behaving like this.' That's when I want to run out of church and get away from everyone, but my role compels me to stay. I'm supposed to be the sorted one – the one that helps other people with their problems. Being at church should be the highlight of my week, but sometimes I dread it.

Being part of a close community makes a situation like childlessness very obvious, particularly a community such as a church where people are used to chatting about the ups and downs of their lives over coffee. It makes us vulnerable in ways that we may find intolerable at times. We wonder whether we should talk about it or not, whether people have the time. We worry that they might say the wrong things. There are only so many times that you can find yourself close to tears in a public place before resolving to clam up completely.

Shaken faith

When we asked people to tell us their story, they often wanted to write about the times when they struggled in their faith.

It sometimes takes longer than we expect to come to terms with what God is doing in our lives. Infertility can bring such disillusionment and disappointment that people can lose sight of who God is and what he is doing in their lives. This might be through thinking that a God who allows such pain cannot love them, or through a dullness that causes them over time to stop going to church, meeting with Christian friends, reading the Bible and praying. However, many men and women can witness to the great strength and perspective that they have received as a result of their distress.

Lucy

Will God give me a baby? I don't know, but I know that he will not put me in a situation I can't handle, and he will take care of me. For now, I'm trying to focus on the good in this seemingly bad situation.

Amy

Where is God in all of this pain? He is right beside me – I have found it hard to feel that he is there at times, but I have learnt that it is not wise always to believe my feelings. Instead, I trust that he is the same faithful and loving God who doesn't change.

SECTION 1:

WHERE IS GOD IN ALL THIS PAIN?

This first section begins with a series of questions that many people in the midst of this experience find themselves asking about God and his purposes for us. As Christians, we want to know what is going on behind the scenes, aware that there is a spiritual dimension to what is happening to us. We also want to recognize that God has the power and the ability to change things. We tend to find ourselves asking why he gives good things to some people and why he denies them to others. Our questions may be prompted both by the accounts of people's lives in the Bible and by the stories we see around us.

But we realize that, for some, these questions may simply not be on the agenda at the moment. If not, then feel free to skip this section, or to come back to it at a later time. There are others who may find themselves weighed down and confused by their current understanding of God. We hope that, by including a detailed examination of these questions, we can point to the bigger picture that is set out for us clearly in the Bible, where we find the place of infertility within God's purposes.

We do not wish to say, 'All you need to do is to understand the Bible better', as if a head knowledge is the only solution to our times of difficulty. At times of deep sadness, we need to mourn with each other and provide comfort through being loving and caring. Even so, we still believe that God works through his Word to bring us an understanding of his will in our hearts. Paul had this desire for Christian believers when he wrote to them in their testing times: 'Since the day we heard about you, we have not stopped praying for you and asking God to fill you with the knowledge of his will through all spiritual wisdom and understanding' (Colossians 1:9).

Paul's words bring these two needs together: the need for personal care and love and the need for growing understanding of what God is doing. Yet even though we may 'know' these things, we still struggle to accept and trust God's purposes. Understanding doesn't necessarily bring relief. But our hope is that the material in this section, over time, will be a means that God uses to restore and strengthen your hope in him.

2 Why me?

Trudy

I was thirty-two when we got married, and was already (in my eyes)
fast ascending, if not quite over, the proverbial hill. We'd discussed
having children during our marriage preparation classes at church
– it was a 'given' really: you had an engagement, you had a wedding,
you had a baby. Motherhood was something I desired very much, and
when nothing happened I was devastated. We had an assortment of
tests . . . the verdict was soon delivered: no reason for our infertility
could be found. This was our new 'given' – we might never be
parents. We had some treatments which were unsuccessful, and
emotionally draining each time they failed. At times the grief was
intense and I would go up to my room and howl and weep.

The feelings experienced by men and women in response to
childlessness are wide ranging and complex, both in intensity
and time frame. Some couples 'feel it' more than others.
Although it is important honestly to acknowledge our grief
and disappointment, this can be hard to do. Sometimes
identifying these feelings to oneself is hard enough. Talking
about them to others, or seeing them in print, is even harder

because then it makes them 'real'. But to pretend that these feelings aren't there would be dishonest.

More questions than answers

Why do we want and hope to be parents so intensely? Why do we grieve so deeply when we cannot have children? For those of us who are Christians, this line of questioning soon leads to God himself. Why is God letting this happen to me? Is it my fault? How does the Bible help me to understand my frustration? We don't have definitive answers to these questions, but it is helpful to look at the pointers given in the book of Genesis. There we begin to see what sort of life God purposed for us in the first place, and there we begin to understand why we don't experience that sort of life any more.

What sort of life did God create me for?

When God created the heavens and the earth, he had generous plans for humankind. When we read Genesis chapter 1, we discover a way of living that God himself wanted us to enjoy.

A life of good things . . .

The idea that God wants us to enjoy a life full of good things sometimes comes as a bit of a shock to people! He is often wrongly thought of as miserly and stingy, unwilling that we should have anything wonderful. If we have ever had this view of God, we only have to look at the beginning of Genesis to see that this simply isn't true. In fact, the very first words of the Bible tell us how wrong we are to think that he withholds good things from us. We are told that the earth was formless and dark (Genesis 1:2). After God has spoken his commands, it is bursting with light and life. It is abundant, beautiful, rich and lush, and everything has its right place in the order of things.

God declares his creation to be 'very good' (Genesis 1:31), because everything works according to how he has planned it. He has, in his goodness and generosity, freely given humankind a wonderful world, packed full of potential and promise.[1]

. . . but where is God's generosity evident today?

Amy

The constant waves of emotion from hope to despair are too much; the disappointment is too crushing. The humiliation of being asked whether my husband and I have children is too shameful. Being told by my doctor that it is not impossible but very unlikely that I will ever get pregnant is too hurtful. I don't do 'possible' or uncertainty. I'm a 'definite' or 'guarantee' kind of person. Where is my God in all of this pain?

Stacey

I find my own inability to get things done at the same rate or with the same efficiency as I did before really frustrating, because I think if I'm not going to have children then I'd like to make the most of the time that I have. I find this confusing because I want to be productive, but I find myself literally incapable of it.

These words echo the great sadness of men and women who see that their lives are empty of the kinds of good things that are offered in Genesis 1. Their bodies are not 'very good' by any stretch of the imagination, because they fail to do the job that God designed fertile bodies to do.

Genesis explains that after the man and woman fall out with God, their lives begin to miss out on the good things that he gave them because the relationship that they had with him and that gave them so much blessing is now in tatters. The garden where they enjoyed so much life and purpose is now completely inaccessible (Genesis 3:23–24). They begin to suffer in many ways as a result. Life from then on is full of difficulty, because it is painful and they are on their own. However hard they would work, there would always be unfulfilled frustrations.

Elspeth

When we started to 'try' for children, I changed jobs so that I was nearer work. I stepped down from a management position and cut down my hours so that I could be ready to leave my job to have children without causing too much disruption. Having children was now my purpose in life. Everything else would have to come later. So when it took longer than we expected, I felt increasingly less useful and less valuable to the world around me. In retrospect, I think it showed up my need to find purpose in my relationship with God rather than in what he wanted me to do in life.

King Solomon, the writer of Ecclesiastes, would agree. He had everything that he could possibly want: power, wisdom and riches.

> Yet when I surveyed all that my hands had done
> and what I had toiled to achieve,
> everything was meaningless, a chasing after the wind;
> nothing was gained under the sun.
> (Ecclesiastes 2:11)

Intensely frustrated

If we understand the consequences of the fall in Genesis 3, then we will consider it inevitable that our childlessness will be marked by deep frustration. There may be little obvious potential or promise in this situation. We may be tempted to think that infertility is just another problem that the human race will eventually solve. Sadly, it is a permanent feature of human existence. There may be advances in medicine that enable us to have a clearer view of the exact problem and even to help us in certain situations. But the problem of infertility will never completely go away.

Stacey

As a woman, I feel totally unproductive. I thought that I would have children and spend my life looking after them. Now I know we can't ever have our own biological children. What am I supposed to do now? Some people suggest that maybe I should throw myself into a more highbrow career, but I want to carry on supporting my husband and being there for him. All the other women who do that seem to have children.

If you have been wanting to have children for a while, then you will know full well that no-one should assume that it will be easy. Sometimes marriage preparation courses include something about infertility, but most leave it out. Stacey added,

When women talk about leaving off having children for a few years, I want to shake them and tell them to get on with it, because it may not happen when you want it to.

So whose fault is it?

The accounts of the creation and the fall in the Bible tell us that we are not to blame. Our spouse is not to blame. Our parents are not to blame. There is no point in trying to point the finger. The occurrences of infertility, the death of a womb or the absence of mature sperm are part of the frustration that creation has been subjected to. Knowing this doesn't necessarily make it any easier to bear, but it may stop us tormenting ourselves with a false guilt.

We expect more than childlessness. We expect fertility and life, children and a happy future. These expectations are chiselled into our very being. But the reality is that we have less. The reality is that we may be frustrated beyond words, blocked at every turn and denied what we most desire.

Wanting children – selfish?

One of the ways in which we were originally designed was with a default setting that saw having children as being a good and desirable goal. That is how God made us. That is what we were created to expect. It is not just for the personal pleasure of humanity, but something that God has asked us to do.

We are told that God's purpose was for man and woman to 'Be fruitful and increase in number; fill the earth and subdue it . . .' (Genesis 1:28). We were to have children in just the same way as the animals, fish and birds did. The man and woman were equally tasked in the job of producing great numbers of people and in ruling over everything on the earth together.

Trevor

In our plans for the future we assumed we would have children. After getting married, we were far more concerned about contraception than anything else. It's laughable when you see what we teach our teenagers in sex education classes; we tell them that the first time you have sex with anyone you'll probably get yourself or the other person pregnant. Realizing we couldn't have children made a mockery of my expectations and dreams. It blew my mind. I'd planned out the rest of my life; I'll do this, then do that. The one thing I didn't have on the plan was infertility. I thought that it was a godly desire to have children and I found myself asking, 'How does that fit into God's control over my life?' God has taught us that the expectations we have are not always his plan.

How does God expect me to cope?

When God created man from the dust of the earth in Genesis 2, he was frail. He had life only because God in his goodness had decided to give it to him, breathing life into him so that he could live. Our very lives are given to us by God and he asks us to recognize our dependency on him. When Jesus told his followers to be like the little children who wanted to come and sit with him, he was pointing out that they needed to have the same unquestioning dependence and trust that those children showed in him: 'I tell you the truth, anyone who will not receive the kingdom of God like a little child will never enter it' (Luke 18:17). This response of dependency was immediately contrasted with that of the rich ruler. He was not able to show the same level of reliance on Jesus as the children. When Jesus asked him to sell everything he had and to follow him, 'he became very sad, because he was a man of great wealth' (18:23). The place of God as the one we trust and depend on at all times and in every way is quickly replaced by anything else that gives us security.

Hard to trust

We find the call to dependency on God deeply difficult. Our world tells us to be confidently independent of God, to stand on our own two feet, to create opportunities for ourselves and make things happen in our own strength. But as soon as Adam and Eve had decided to operate independently of God, they did not experience confidence and resolve. Instead, they were full of fear:

> Then the man and his wife heard the sound of the LORD God as he was walking in the garden in the cool of the day, and they hid from the LORD God among the trees of the garden. But the LORD God called to the man, 'Where are you?'
>
> He answered, 'I heard you in the garden, and I was afraid because I was naked; so I hid.'
>
> (Genesis 3:8–10)

How about that for feeling vulnerable! It is the complete opposite to dependency. There was the Lord God, walking in the garden, down on their level, wanting to be with them in the relationship that he had established with them. There they were, desperately trying to get away from him because they could not face him as they were.

They had been suspicious that God was holding something back from them and so they ate the fruit of the tree that had been forbidden, so that they might be 'like God, knowing good and evil' (Genesis 3:5). Sin has completely spoilt their view of God. Rather than seeing him as the Creator who has blessed them with the fullness of life, they see him as a tyrant who should be feared.[2]

It is now in our nature to want to feel that we are in control over our own lives, rather than letting God be in control. We find it so hard to let him carry out the purposes that he has for us. As Nate's experience shows, we tend to shut God out of the plans we have for the future and put ourselves in control instead.

Nate

*When we had been checked out medically and found out that I was
the one with the problem, I behaved like a pouty little child. I looked
for the things that would benefit me in the situation, like having more
sex more often. Even then I was emotionally absent. I made sex and
getting pregnant into an idol, and I thought that I was the only one
who could solve this problem. As well as trying to shut out God,
I also shut out my wife. It led to feelings of guilt, disappointment
and sadness. My inner macho male felt completely inadequate, and
I was in a bad place. I knew deep down that I hadn't done anything
to deserve God's blessing.*

What do I have from God?

Frustrations today make God's abundant generosity in the
original creation seem a long way away. We may think that
without children there are few good things in our lives and
little evidence of God's kindness to us. When Jesus talks to
people about God's generosity, he speaks to those who may
have very little in the world's eyes: 'Do not worry, saying,
"What shall we eat?" or "What shall we drink?" or "What
shall we wear?" For the pagans run after all these things, and
your heavenly Father knows that you need them' (Matthew
6:31–32).

He wants people to see God's generosity in terms of what
they have in knowing him, rather in terms of what they do
not have. The people Jesus is talking to here probably struggle
to make ends meet. For them, the issues are money, clothes,
food and drink – things that are good in themselves, but which
can also carry us away from God in a tangle of worry and
obsession. Jesus wants his followers to see God's goodness
and generosity in spiritual riches, which are on permanent
offer to everyone.

I wonder if we can transfer this understanding of God's generosity to our own lives. Can we take Jesus' lead and try to nurture our understanding that God really *is* good? That he really *does* want us to have good things: good things that he has already given us in abundance? Those things may not include children at this moment in time, but it doesn't mean that God is mean or miserly. God asks that in our experience of struggling with infertility we seek potential and promise in him.

Why is this happening to me?

Our experience of frustration in the face of suffering is not happening to us just because we are Christians. This is happening because everyone has universally fallen out with the God who made us. We suffer in our own personal ways as a result. Even without the problem of infertility, we will find it hard to discover fulfilment and purpose in our lives. Our frustration is inevitable and we are right to expect more, but the reality is that we have less.

3 Will God give me a child?

Jacqui

Hearing about people who have had babies just depresses me. I genuinely find it difficult to understand the basis on which God gives children to some people and not to others. I believe that God is all-powerful and that he loves me. Why doesn't he show his power and his love in making it possible for us to have a baby? If I believe that 'in all things God works for the good of those who love him', then what is the good that will come out of this situation? People say that they are sure that God will give us a baby and they tell us that they are praying we will have one. How do they know? Will their prayers make any difference?

God has a plan for us

If you find that Jacqui's frustration mirrors your own, you bear witness to the fact that many childless people struggle with this craving to know God's mind and purpose in their situation. We want to know what God has in store for us. Whenever we ask questions about God's plan for our lives, it is a good idea to look at the Bible, since that is where God's plan for his people is explained.

> *Jacqui*
> *The truth is that I don't see the point in reading about any of the women in the Bible who are infertile. I don't want to torture myself by reading about God's gift to them when he hasn't given me that same gift.*

We may be reluctant to look at the accounts of childlessness in the Bible because most infertile couples there are eventually given babies. Even so, these stories are there to teach us something about God himself: to show us his basis for giving a childless couple a baby and to show us why it is important that he does that; to show that we actually benefit today from his giving them that baby. Then we will be equipped to learn wonderful things from these people about who God is and how he works, rather than end up resenting them.

Our greatest need

> *Jacqui*
> *When people try to help me to keep going, they sometimes talk about Abraham. They suggest that since Abraham had faith, I should too. They tell me not to give up because God could give me a baby as well.*

Some Christians will use Abraham as an example of having faith when you're infertile. Perhaps this is because the arrival of Isaac in Abraham's household is such an unlikely and joyful event, and people would love that to happen for us too. They want us to believe that God can do the impossible – to believe that God could do this for me too.

> Sarah said, 'God has brought me laughter, and everyone who
> hears about this will laugh with me.' And she added, 'Who
> would have said to Abraham that Sarah would nurse children?
> Yet I have borne him a son in his old age.'
> (Genesis 21:6–7)

But a closer reading of Abraham's situation helps us to understand that we cannot compare ourselves with him. This is a unique event in God's plan. Sadly, it does not give us any reason to conclude that today's childless couples can also expect that God will give them a child.

Abraham and Sarah

The horror of Abraham's situation was that Sarah's childlessness was preventing God's people from coming into being. For Christians, Abraham's story is vital. Without him, there would be no line of descendants to lead to Christ, God's means of salvation. It is this line of descendants that comes under threat when Abraham doesn't have children.

It wasn't a short period of childlessness, either. Abraham was already seventy-five when God first promised that a nation would come from him (Genesis 12:2), about eighty-six when his wife told him to sleep with Hagar (Genesis 16:16) and a hundred years old when Sarah finally gave birth to Isaac (Genesis 21:5). That is twenty-four years of waiting, following on *after* the lifetime that they had already experienced without having any children.

Paul discusses Abraham's faith with regard to waiting for children in the New Testament book of Romans:

> Without weakening in his faith, he faced the fact that his body
> was as good as dead – since he was about a hundred years

old – and that Sarah's womb was also dead. Yet he did not
waver through unbelief regarding the promise of God, but
was strengthened in his faith and gave glory to God, being
fully persuaded that God had power to do what he had
promised.
(Romans 4:19–21)

Abraham didn't have the ability himself to produce children.
He and Sarah were old and barren. But in their old age they
had faith in who God was and in what he was able to do.

Abraham knew that God could deliver on his promises

[Abraham] is our father in the sight of God, in whom he
believed – the God who gives life to the dead and calls things
that are not as though they were.

Against all hope, Abraham in hope believed and so became
the father of many nations, just as it had been said to him,
'So shall your offspring be.'
(Romans 4:17–18)

Abraham was putting his faith in what God had told him
would happen. God had said that he would be the father of
many nations, so Abraham was right to trust that God would
make that happen. After all, the God he knew has limitless
power. He was 'fully persuaded that God had power to do
what he had promised'. He trusted that God could give 'life
to the dead' and that he could call 'things that are not as
though they were'. We are not told exactly what Abraham's
frame of logic was, but we can assume that he knew how the
world began. If God could create the universe out of nothing,
then he could bring about a child in an empty womb. If

he could form Adam and Eve out of the dust of the earth, he could make another person without needing fertile parents. God promised Abraham that he would be the father of nations, and Abraham knew that God had the power to deliver on that promise, however unlikely it seemed.

Isaac's birth meant many things

Happily, the birth of Isaac proves that God is able to fulfil his promises, no matter what. He promised to give Abraham descendants. Well, he did that. He also promised to bless all nations through his offspring. From the viewpoint of the New Testament, we now know that this offspring is Jesus. We know that this blessing is one of forgiveness and eternal life: peace with God, no matter what our background. God in his goodness teaches us that the main purpose of Isaac's birth was not to relieve Abraham and Sarah of their childlessness. It was to provide me today with the possibility of a relationship with God. This is incredible and brilliant news. It puts the gift of a child to these people into perspective. It shows how good and faithful God was in his actions of giving them a baby, and how good and faithful he was to me.

Ancient Israel and infertility stress

The gift of a child to infertile couples in the Old Testament is shown to be even more amazing when we find out a little bit about their culture. Like any other ancient civilization, not to mention some developing countries today, it was important to keep your land and your family name. This was particularly true for a small nation like Israel, which would be under threat from surrounding countries.

Children provided practical help in working the land and providing for their parents in their old age. They were also your own personal army, helping to fight off your enemies. Having large numbers of children was of practical import-ance, which is why sons were synonymous with prosperity and success.

> Like arrows in the hands of a warrior
>> are sons born in one's youth.
> Blessed is the man
>> whose quiver is full of them.
> They will not be put to shame
>> when they contend with their enemies in the gate.
> (Psalm 127:4–5)

This concern is reflected in special laws that God gave to his people, such as the law of the kinsman-redeemer, which we see at work in the story of Ruth and Boaz.

> Then Boaz announced to the elders and all the people, 'Today you are witnesses that I have bought from Naomi all the property of Elimelech, Kilion and Mahlon. I have also acquired Ruth the Moabitess, Mahlon's widow, as my wife, in order to maintain the name of the dead with his property, so that his name will not disappear from among his family or from the town records. Today you are witnesses!'
> (Ruth 4:9–10)

Those without children in these ancient times faced a host of issues that we know little about in our world of pension plans, nursing homes, benefits and emergency services. The gravity of an infertile couple's situation meant that God's grace was all the more wonderful when a baby was born.

So when we consider God's will for our lives and wonder whether or not he will give us children, we can say with confidence that his first priority is our relationship with him. When we see him at work in the lives of Abraham and Sarah, we see him at work in our own lives too – not to give us a child, but to bring us back to him.

Other infertile couples in the Bible

So far we have mentioned only Abraham. We have not yet thought about the parents of Joseph, Samson, Samuel and John the Baptist, who were all unable to have children until they came along. The Old Testament examples here were all so important that they are directly referred to alongside Abraham as heroes of the faith in Hebrews 11. Each one played a part in revealing God's plan of salvation at significant points in Israel's history. Each was involved in kicking the ball along towards God's goal: the goal that anybody from any nation could be 'made right with God' through Jesus.

Joseph, born to Rachel and Jacob, was to be a saviour of God's people. When he rose to power in Egypt, he was able to house and feed all of Israel throughout many years of famine. It was while they lived in the land of Egypt for 400 years that they grew from twelve families numbering seventy people into twelve tribes, forming the great nation that God had promised Abraham: 'Now Joseph and all his brothers and all that generation died, but the Israelites were fruitful and multiplied greatly and became exceedingly numerous, so that the land was filled with them' (Exodus 1:6–7).

Samson, born to the wife of Manoah, was a judge over Israel, saving them from their enemies, the Philistines.

Samuel, born to Elkanah and Hannah, was to become the prophet who spoke God's wisdom to Israel's godless king, Saul.

John the Baptist, born to Elizabeth and Zechariah, was to be the messenger to go ahead and prepare the way for Jesus as he led people to repentance and pointed to the arrival of the long-awaited Christ.

These stories of infertility are there to show us that throughout the time before Jesus' birth, God was in control. In one sense, the Old Testament is all about the long wait for a baby. But we are not like Abraham and Sarah, or any other of these infertile couples. The baby that everyone had been waiting for is Jesus and he has been born. God can of course work miracles and do amazing things in people's lives. But he no longer needs to demonstrate his power through overcoming infertility, because he has demonstrated his power once and for all in the death and resurrection of Jesus:

> Praise be to the God and Father of our Lord Jesus Christ! In his great mercy he has given us new birth into a living hope through the resurrection of Jesus Christ from the dead, and into an inheritance that can never perish, spoil or fade.
>
> (1 Peter 1:3–4a)

God's people may go on having children, but the emphasis is now on the spiritual new life that will continue beyond their death. We can see that the magnitude of God's love is demonstrated once and for all as he makes peace with us, individually, through the death of his Son.

Salvation *since* Jesus: spiritual new birth

Trevor and Stacey
One Sunday at our church, the service began with a birth announcement. The baby had arrived the night before. There was

a photo of the baby, which was projected on to the overhead screen.
There was mass cooing and aahing. There had been a birth the
weekend before, too, and so a second photo of an equally cute baby
followed. Cue more excited noises from the congregation. We have
recently heard that we are unable to have children. Of course we
want to rejoice with those who are rejoicing, but it took us by
surprise. Church is the only place where we can rejoice about
spiritual new birth with our fellow believers, and we wondered
whether the news of physical births should have taken up quite
so much time.

The New Testament part of the Bible is no longer preoccupied
with physical births and genealogies. God's plan for a nation
of people is no longer concerned with the continuation of
one people group or culture. The baby has arrived. He will
complete everything that has been started. Now that anyone
can be made right with God, the type of birth that he is
concerned with is spiritual birth.

> Jesus declared, 'I tell you the truth, no-one can see the
> kingdom of God unless he is born again.'
> 'How can a man be born when he is old?' Nicodemus asked,
> 'Surely he cannot enter a second time into his mother's womb
> to be born!'
> Jesus answered, 'I tell you the truth, no-one can enter the
> kingdom of God unless he is born of water and the Spirit.
> Flesh gives birth to flesh, but the Spirit gives birth to spirit.'
> (John 3:3–6)

Those who have been born twice can enter the kingdom of
God. So the books of the New Testament focus on bringing
new birth and new life to people through Jesus. Although our
physical life will end one day, our spiritual lives will not. The

really exciting news that our church leaders should be bursting to tell us, and the news that we should be most eager to hear, is the news of new spiritual life in Christ.

We see this joy at spiritual new birth in the first words uttered by Zechariah, the father of John the Baptist, when his child is born. In personal terms, we might have thought that the birth of his son would be a great opportunity to thank God for blessing him and his wife with a child after a long life of childlessness. Everyone is preoccupied by what name he will give the child, but he only wants to speak of what God is doing to fulfil his promises and save his people. He says:

> Praise be to the Lord, the God of Israel,
>> because he has come and has redeemed his people.
> He has raised up a horn of salvation for us
>> in the house of his servant David
> (as he said through his holy prophets of long ago).
> (Luke 1:68–70)

God's promises to us

We have not been given the promise by God that we will have a child. We have been given other promises, though. We have been promised that we have been given new birth, new life, by God through faith in the death of Jesus. This reassures us that God is for us, whatever our circumstances.

> The words 'it was credited to him' were written not for [Abraham] alone, but also for us, to whom God will credit righteousness – for us who believe in him who raised Jesus our Lord from the dead. He was delivered over to death for our sins and was raised to life for our justification.
> (Romans 4:23–25)

So when we consider what God's plan might be for us, when we wonder whether we can have any certainty that he might give us a baby, we need to remember the goal of God's plan. We can look at the Bible and find out what God's will is for our lives. His will is that we might be made right with God and given our own new life through Jesus' death and resurrection. How extraordinary that he used infertile couples and their longing for children back then as he worked out his plan for us today.

4 Childless – *and* blessed?

Kate

As a young child growing up with a brother and parents in a comfortable home in a small market town, I used to dream of being married and having four sons. I was born with a congenital abnormality which I subsequently came to realize also meant that it was unlikely (but not impossible) that I would be able to have children. It took me until my mid-forties to be able to say, 'Sadly I do not have children, although I would have loved to have them.'

Annie and Jack

Many people talk about children as a gift from God, and how much they are blessed by having them. Sometimes, a feeling can come about that, maybe, I wasn't blessed as much.

Much as we might long to have children, we can see that God does not promise for certain that we will have any. We cannot hold him to a promise that he never made in the first place. We understand that his promise to Abraham is unique.

But now, this topic of 'blessing' moves us on to another area of the Bible that is frequently misused in the counselling of infertile couples. We can see how easy it is to convey the wrong understanding of 'blessing' when we talk about how 'blessed' people are to have children. Annie and Jack's conclusion that they weren't 'blessed as much' shows us that. Our choice of the word 'blessing' can communicate a variety of messages. It might be the message that we are being rewarded for obedience or, conversely, that we are being punished for disobedience.

Blessings and curses

We can find ourselves reading the Old Testament book of Deuteronomy and discovering that children were promised as a blessing because of obedience to God:

> If you fully obey the LORD your God and carefully follow all his commands that I give you today, the LORD your God will set you high above all the nations on earth. All these blessings will come upon you and accompany you if you obey the LORD your God:
>
> > You will be blessed in the city and blessed in the country. The fruit of your womb will be blessed.
>
> (Deuteronomy 28:1–4a)

Some Christians wrongly conclude from these verses that if we do not experience these blessings then it might be that we are experiencing some sort of curse from God instead.

Craig
A friend who is a really switched-on Christian was thinking out loud when he was talking to me, and said, 'Why do you not think that being infertile is God cursing you? That's what it says in the Old Testament.'

Under God's curse?

In the Old Testament we do indeed read about curses that Israel will face if it fails to be obedient to God's commands. These lists of curses include the condition of infertility.

Paul tells the Galatians about this, quoting the Old Testament: 'All who rely on observing the law are under a curse, for it is written: "Cursed is everyone who does not continue to do everything written in the Book of the Law"' (Galatians 3:10).

It is interesting to note here that infertile people cannot be singled out as those who might be 'under a curse', since it is applied to anyone failing to obey God. That covers everybody! Paul goes on to show us definitively that we cannot possibly be under a curse. When Christ died on the cross, he was cursed instead of us. We do indeed deserve it for failing to obey God, but Jesus took the punishment of that curse so that we did not have to: 'Christ redeemed us from the curse of the law by becoming a curse for us, for it is written: "Cursed is everyone who is hung on a tree"' (Galatians 3:13).

I hope that this will give you the confidence to answer anyone foolish enough to consider that this might be the case for you. When we are weakened emotionally, it is sometimes hard to be convinced of this truth, but we hope that God will reassure you of his great love for you in Jesus.

Although God's blessings can include children . . .

Many would describe the following as signs of God's blessing: good health, a happy marriage, good relationships, a successful job or career, children, a comfortable home, good food, happy holidays. All of these are certainly 'good', and we should be continually thankful to God for them. So, yes, children are a sign of God's goodness and generosity now.

. . . they are not the way in which God has proved his love for us

It is easy to agree that these are things that we should be thankful for. It is harder to work out why, if God loves to give good things to his people, he is not giving us the children we desire, out of compassion for us. We struggle with feelings that God can't see how hard this is. We feel that we are not blessed.

The problem arises when we start to think of all of these things as conditional upon our being good. We may start to see them as an expectation or a 'right', especially if we've been good, faithful Christians. We may begin to view them as signs of God's favour with us. The consequence of thinking like this can be that when I don't experience these things, or if they are taken away from me, I think God is not 'blessing' me. I feel that God doesn't love me. It is sometimes extremely hard to identify God's goodness in our lives when we are over-whelmed by the absence of the one thing that we really desire.

Catherine

I remember desperately wanting the ear of my minister on one occasion. She was obviously very stretched, having two young children, one of whom needed to go to the doctor. So, she suggested that instead of coming to her house for tea and a chat, I accompanied them to the doctor. I really had only half her ear! She asked me a number of questions, while dealing with her children, I forget what about, and I guess my answers were all pretty negative. Eventually she said to me 'So what good things are happening in your life, Catherine?' That really hurt! It was all I could do to draw on my head knowledge and let

her know that through the lows, I knew God was with me and holding
me. Even my heart was struggling to believe it by this time.

Emily
As a Christian facing the fact that I wasn't able to have children,
I found myself feeling guilty that I wasn't trusting God enough. I
know how much God has given me in my life. I am so grateful for my
husband. I have loving parents and a great job that I enjoy. My health
is good in all other areas apart from this. But none of that seems to
count for anything any more. I find it so hard to work out why this
feels as bad as it does. I love God and I'm so grateful for Jesus and all
that he has done for me. I want to serve him and live for him, but I
feel so paralysed by my inability to get pregnant.

Both Catherine and Emily already know they are blessed. Yet
they still reflect a real desire to know in their hearts what it
means to be blessed by God when they are denied a good thing
that they know he gives to others. The challenge for them and
for us is how we can know God's blessing at this time as a
reality that goes deeper than head knowledge: a blessing that
encourages us to be dependent on God in this particular area
of our lives.

Every spiritual blessing

Amy
God is perfect love – his love for me is so great, it is beyond compare
and comprehension. It was so great that he gave his most precious
thing, his Son, to die for me. Who am I to understand a God like
this? His ways are not my ways. So will I ever be a mother? It's
possible. Does God have a plan for me that is ultimately the best
it could be? Definitely. Will he stay beside me and not leave me?
That is a guarantee.

Amy knows that her status before God has been changed by Jesus' death and resurrection. She knows that her acceptance by God is not conditional upon obeying his commands. He accepts her because she has been made right with him when Jesus died on the cross. She knows that his love for her and his control over her life extend beyond mere fact, and we see God sustaining her deep down in her grief. It would be hard to say that Amy wasn't blessed.

The proof of God's love for me is not that he gives me children. The proof of his love for me is that he sent Jesus, his only Son, to die for me. For the Christian today, this is marvellous news. Knowing this should help to guard against seeking some kind of assurance that God shows his love for me by giving me a child: 'Praise be to the God and Father of our Lord Jesus Christ, who has blessed us in the heavenly realms with every spiritual blessing in Christ' (Ephesians 1:3).

As we read on in Ephesians, we can see that the main blessing available to all who believe now is forgiveness for sins through the death and resurrection of Jesus. As Ephesians 1 unfolds, Paul illustrates what this blessing fully encompasses now and in the future. We are chosen to be holy and blameless, adopted as sons, and we have received free grace, redemption and forgiveness of sins (Ephesians 1:4–8). And in Romans, the blessings given through Christ are peace and reconciliation with God (Romans 5:1, 11).

By dying and being raised to life, Jesus dealt with God's anger at our sin, making all his promised blessings possible. We live in between times now, and we experience the effects of a decaying, frustrated, fallen world (of which infertility is one). These effects may make us lose sight of God's amazing blessings. But we can be certain of our future adoption as God's children because we have every spiritual blessing in Christ. After a long period of frustration and pain, Christine concludes that she has indeed been fully blessed in Christ.

Christine

I now feel very blessed by God, even though we have no family. My husband and I have many friends, young and old, and we are doing what we hope are useful things in a community that we are growing to love. It has been a twenty-year process!

Blessed more than Abraham!

Amazingly, the blessings and promises that God gave to Abraham are spiritual blessings and promises to us, too: to all those who, like Abraham, have faith in God's promises to them. '[Christ] redeemed us in order that the blessing given to Abraham might come to the Gentiles through Christ Jesus, so that by faith we might receive the promise of the Spirit' (Galatians 3:14).

We are the ones who have benefited from everything that Abraham had to face. If we consider that he was blessed, then we need to realize that we have been blessed far more than he ever was. We have Jesus. Luke records a sermon given to the Jews by Paul in Acts 13, where Paul shows that the resurrection of Christ links back to God's promises to Israel:

We tell you the good news: What God promised our fathers he has fulfilled for us, their children, by raising up Jesus. As it is written in the second Psalm:

'You are my Son;
today I have become your Father.'

The fact that God raised him from the dead, never to decay, is stated in these words:

> 'I will give you the holy and sure blessings promised to David.'
> (Acts 13:32–34)

Do you still trust in Christ? You are blessed. Are you still looking forward to the day when Christ will return to bring all things under his head? You are blessed. Do you still trust in the glory that will be revealed in you and are you waiting eagerly for your adoption as God's child? You are blessed.

This still feels awful

This truth is not always going to slap a smile on your face and put a spring in your step. We may be able to agree with everything in this chapter and still feel an emotional wreck.

Trevor
Feelings often don't match up with what we can 'know theologically'. They may still mislead us, even when we know what the truth is. This can have the effect of making us feel guilty and not very good Christians, when things that we know don't seem to have an impact on our emotions and behaviour. It doesn't mean we aren't Christians, but we need to remember that our feelings are a poor guide to the truth.

God created us to be emotional creatures, and part of our make-up is our acute awareness of pain. What does it look like to confront this pain and to keep going?

5 This hurts

Craig

When we hit problems, we were blunt with God. We asked him 'What is the logic in this? What are you doing? You give us great gifts and talents and then stop us from being able to use them as parents. You give children to sixteen-year-olds who can't look after them. What possible good can come from not giving us a baby?' Looking back, we are grateful that we had been taught really well from the Bible about suffering. If we hadn't known that suffering is a reality in the lives of Christians and not a sign of spiritual failure, then I think we would have been completely shipwrecked.

Feeling incomplete

If we struggle with infertility, it may be that we experience an inner conflict that is hard to understand. We may feel satisfied with the life that God has given us in every area except this one. We may be consumed with a hunger and desire for having children that makes us feel selfish and guilty. We can't understand why this particular thing that is lacking in our life is causing us such grief.

Understanding creation helps us to realize that we are right to want children. It is God's idea. We are wired up that way. It helps us to understand that our longing for children is right and good and is not fundamentally selfish. It is nothing to be ashamed of.

In fact the Bible shows us how deeply God understands this desire. The author of Proverbs articulates this craving for children:

> There are three things that are never satisfied,
>   four that never say, 'Enough!':
> the grave, the barren womb,
>   land, which is never satisfied with water,
>   and fire, which never says, 'Enough!'
> (Proverbs 30:15b–16)

You get close to understanding the longing of a childless couple for a baby when you think about these other things. Think about those TV images of raging forest fires that we see every summer, consuming everything in their paths, or the famine-struck desert on the news, ready to soak up any amount of water you could pour on it. They are images for us to ponder on so that we might have an insight into the psychology of infertility. Facing childlessness can be a consuming, hungry and ravaging experience, which can threaten to overpower the strongest faith.

Singled out?

Lucy
*As we asked our family and friends for prayers and support, I
began to feel the weight of the reality of our situation; every time
I admitted it to someone, I admitted to myself that we might never be*

parents. Once the reality of the loss and grief set in, I cried a lot and
began to ask why God gave us this struggle. Is it to prove that he
really is in control? Is it because my husband and I are not mature
enough to raise a child? Is it to teach us another lesson? I wondered
whether, if we had lived our life differently, God would have changed
his plans for us.

After Eleanor and I had given a talk on infertility to a group
of Christian women, someone asked a question along the
lines of Lucy's thoughts: 'How do I cope when I feel singled
out by God for this trial?' Behind this question we were sure
was a real tension – how do you square your personal pain
with your belief that everything in this life is sovereignly
ordained by God? Does God knowingly inflict this suffering?

This is a hard one. It's fine to believe that God is sovereign
when good things come. But infertility? If we are to be true
to the Bible, we have to take heed of what we read, even when
it feels uncomfortable. It was hard to answer this question
compassionately without sounding callous, because we are
told in Isaiah that God brings good things *and* calamity.
'I know, O LORD, that your laws are righteous, and in faithfulness you have afflicted me' (Psalm 119:75).

So, in a real sense, we have been singled out for this trial.
My childlessness is not plan B. This is not to say that God gets
some pleasure out of our suffering, but rather that he has a
purpose in ordaining it. As with any suffering, we naturally
would like to be *released* from its pain. We want it to stop. But
there is a sense in which we may never 'get over it', because
the grief of infertility or miscarriage can be a deep, long-lasting
pain. However, we can experience a greater hope, rather than
just bearing the pain more manageably, or trying to understand 'why' this has happened. This side of heaven, we
may never know why we have been given this specific trial.

Our greater hope is that God has a rich purpose for our sufferings.

Belinda

I suffered several miscarriages before a very early menopause. Most occurred early on in the pregnancy, but at least two went to two or three months. Often I echoed the experience of Hannah and other childless women of the Bible: tears, frustration, sorrow, self-pity, even anger – all out of a natural desire that was not met when and how I wanted. Today, looking back, I can honestly say that 'God does all things well'. He's in the business of bringing us closer to himself and helping us to grow in our understanding of what he is like as a loving heavenly Father. His plans for us are so much bigger, better, wider, richer and more adventurous than our own.

Feeling abandoned

What compounds our distress is a feeling of being abandoned and unloved by God. Even when we might know in our heads that this is not true, we still feel far from him. When earnest prayers for a child have not been answered, many experience an absence of peace, strength, courage and joy: 'O God, do not keep silent; be not quiet, O God, be not still' (Psalm 83:1).

It sometimes takes longer than we expect to come to terms with what God is doing in our lives.

How do we bear the silence of God?

David, the chosen king anointed by God to rule the people of Israel, was also someone who at times felt abandoned by God. He cried out in words that Jesus himself used when he was dying on the cross:

My God, my God, why have you forsaken me?
 Why are you so far from saving me,
 so far from the words of my groaning?
O my God, I cry out by day, but you do not answer,
 by night, and am not silent.
(Psalm 22:1–2)

David goes on to speak of God's past actions of rescue
and deliverance and to point to his promises for the future.
God has promised that he will be seen by all to be the
King and Ruler. Everyone will one day bow before him,
the afflicted will eat and be satisfied, and our hearts will live
for ever.

Silent, not absent

For he has not despised or disdained
 the suffering of the afflicted one;
he has not hidden his face from him
 but has listened to his cry for help.
(Psalm 22:24)

God listened to David's cries for help. He has heard yours, too.
He is with you in your isolation.

Helen
After the death of our daughter, a day after she was born at twenty-four weeks' gestation, we know that the Lord suffered with us, drew close to us, upheld and faithfully sustained us each day, each hour, each minute . . .

Jesus used Psalm 22 when he cried out as he was crucified.
He chose to hold firm to God's promises, even though for

him at the time it meant experiencing isolation, darkness and extreme physical suffering while bearing the silence of God. Jesus bore God's silence, knowing that it wasn't the end of the story, and, at his darkest hour, he prayed for God's will to be done, knowing that this alone would bring glory to God: 'Father, the time has come. Glorify your Son, that your Son may glorify you' (John 17:1b).

If you experience God's silence now, pray for this same hope; that God has heard and that his purposes will be accomplished. Psalm 22 ends with this great promise of restoration for God's people as he is glorified:

> The poor will eat and be satisfied;
>   they who seek the LORD will praise him –
>   may your hearts live for ever! . . .
> Posterity will serve him;
>   future generations will be told about the Lord.
> They will proclaim his righteousness
>   to a people yet unborn –
>   for he has done it.
> (Psalm 22:26, 30–31)

God was glorified as Jesus was raised from the dead. This same God hears us, and we will one day praise him again. The hope we can offer to one another is that God has heard us, even if we feel abandoned.

But I feel so angry

Trudy

At times I felt that my prayers bounced off the walls of heaven. I felt angry and abandoned by God: why couldn't he fix it?

Christine

*I have to say that the first few years of my thirties were a very
dark time, with a great many tears shed. For a while I was
very angry with God. But as time went on I realized that he had
other plans for me, and that it was better to be accepting of the
situation and make the best of it. I think this took a long time –
many years.*

The grief of infertility and childlessness will at times result
in feelings of intense anger. This anger may be directed
towards God and towards friends and family who misunder-
stand or who become pregnant. Anger may be accompanied
by irritation when pregnant women complain of illness,
or by impatience when new parents complain of fatigue
and lack of sleep. It causes much internal conflict and soul
searching because it is difficult to square this with the
scriptural advice to rejoice with those who rejoice in Romans
12:15.

It is important to say from the outset that a lack of deep
feeling about infertility would be unusual. It might be worth
articulating what you are angry about. Paul David Tripp
helps to point to the root of our anger: 'It's hard to admit, but
when we are angry we are in reality angry at God. In our
bitterness we summon him to the court of our judgement
and charge him with being unloving, unkind, unfair or
unfaithful.'[1]

In the Bible there seems to be a difference between anger
and sin. In other words, it is possible to be angry and not sinful.
Psalm 4 says, 'In your anger do not sin . . . ' (verse 4). But what
might this look like?

> . . . when you are on your beds,
>   search your hearts and be silent.

Offer right sacrifices
  and trust in the LORD.
(Psalm 4:4–5)

Sin is a refusal to allow God to be God, and wanting to rule your own life in your own way. So when you feel angry, don't give in to feelings of self-pity, harsh words to others, bitterness or hard-heartedness. Ask yourself why you are angry. Tell God you are angry, pray to him for forgiveness where necessary, and ask him to help you trust him and his purposes.

Remembered by God

God has not left us without comfort or hope. He remembers the childless. Nestled within the many promises God makes to his people in Isaiah is a specific future blessing directed to the childless:

. . . a memorial and a name
  better than sons and daughters
. . . an everlasting name
  that will not be cut off.
(Isaiah 56:4–5)

Asking for professional help . . .

It may be that the stresses of our situation develop to a point where we need to ask for help. A study has shown that rates of clinical depression amongst women trying to conceive are the same as for those with heart disease or cancer![2] Ironically, sexual dysfunction for men is another side effect, making it impossible to create the much-needed opportunities for conception. If you suspect that you may be clinically depressed or if you are facing dysfunction, then talk to your doctor about it. He or she can help you to make the right decisions regarding medication and counselling, and may also know of support groups in your local area.

. . . while God is at work within us

Infertility can be a suffering that *doesn't end*. As with any suffering, we naturally would like to be released from it. We want it to stop. But as we mourn in chronic grief, how does God work in us? The authentic Christian response to our suffering through infertility is to trust that God will supply our every need, that he will work through this particular circumstance to make us more like Christ, and will give us the hope of eternity where all suffering will cease. I don't think I can put it better than Sam and Polly's words, which articulate the experience of having a stillborn child:

> We don't pretend to have anything other than general theological answers as to why this should happen, but we tend to say, 'Why not?' And why shouldn't we accept from our heavenly Father, who has given us all things in Christ, the privilege of suffering along with others, especially if it enables us to relate better to them in their suffering? We know that, relatively speaking, we have suffered little; at the same time we also know that our experience has its place in God's good plan for us, and we are content in him.

Reflecting on chapters 2 – 5

Something to read

As you look at the following passages, what sources of strength does God give us in our suffering?

1 Peter 1:6b–7: Why does God send us these trials? What further comfort does Peter offer the suffering Christian in 1 Peter 4:12–19?

2 Corinthians 4:16–17: Where does Paul turn, in his weakness and affliction, in order to give him hope?

2 Corinthians 12:9–10: What is the consequence of Paul's ongoing sufferings?

Something to do

What are the good things that God has given you? Draw up a list or a mind-map with all the 'blessings' that you see in your life. Then read Ephesians 1:3–14 and add to your list all of the spiritual blessings that God has given us. Pray that God will make these blessings more valuable to you than they are already.

A conversation to have

Try to describe what it is like to want children that you cannot have. Ask a friend to listen without wanting to talk about what your next step should be or where you will go from here. Just articulate what it is like for you here and now. It might be helpful for you to use some of the verses quoted in this section as prayers.

For friends and pastors

Don't feel the need to jump in and give hope in the form of theological instruction when you see people caught up emotionally by infertility. Don't be put off-guard by their confusion. Listen to them and pray with them, particularly along the lines of Romans 8 and the experience of living with this intense frustration.

Further reading

John Piper and Justin Taylor, *Suffering and the Sovereignty of God* (Crossway, 2006).
Don Carson, *How Long, O Lord?* (Inter-Varsity Press, 1990).

SECTION 2:

COPING WITH THE STRESS
OF CHILDLESSNESS

6 Who am I, without a family?

Mary

At the time of diagnosis I initially felt quite sensitive about our being a childless married couple in a church that is very family focused. I have felt low and have experienced self-doubt, with so many questions about where not being able to have a family leaves us.

Mary's sensitivity highlights the discomfort and dislocation many childless and single men and women often feel in churches. Our individual identity and role within the church are questioned by the strong emphasis churches place on 'family'. 'Families welcome!' shout the billboards outside. 'Events for families!' scream the fliers. 'How wonderful to celebrate the new addition to the X family!' says the service leader in the church notices. 'Do you have a family?' asks a friendly soul over coffee, who notices that we have no infants attached to our ankles.

The question that is commonly asked is 'If I have no children, do I really belong in this fertile throng of community that is my church?' Before we feel tempted to leave and move to a different service or another, 'family-free' church, we need to ask, 'How does God view families, and how does he include me in his own family? What does it mean to live as part of his family?'

What makes a family?

In the Old Testament, families, or 'households', tended to contain more people than the biologically related parents and children, such as elderly and widowed relatives and servants. The people of Israel were part of one large extended kinship group descended from Abraham. Within this large group were the twelve tribes, according to the twelve sons of Jacob. Within these tribes were the clans, which were made up of a collection of extended family units of relatives and servants which each contained fifteen to twenty-five people. This unit was known as a *bêt 'āb*, which literally translates as 'father's house'.[1]

A new family

Tom
We have a spiritual family to care for and be involved with, which is an enormous blessing.

The New Testament has a view of family based on Christ. This is a revolutionary new definition of family. What Christ's death and resurrection have achieved for the whole of the human race radically redefines who my 'family' is. All Christian believers have the same heavenly Father and are part of the same family. The simple answer to the question 'Do you have a family?' is a resounding 'Yes!' Paul talks to the Ephesian Christians about the great bond that the people of Israel and Gentile (non-Israelite) believers have because of Christ.

> Through the gospel the Gentiles are heirs together with
> Israel, members together of one body, and sharers together
> in the promise of Christ Jesus . . .
>
> For this reason I kneel before the Father, from whom
> his whole family in heaven and on earth derives its
> name.
> (Ephesians 3:6, 14–15)

God is our Father

When we look at who God is and what aspects of his character he has chosen to reveal to us, we see that he longs for us
to know that he is a Father. He has a Son whom he loves – Jesus
Christ, who responds to him in obedi-ence. Jesus frequently
talks to his disciples about his Father:

> As the Father has loved me, so have I loved you. Now remain
> in my love. If you obey my commands, you will remain in my
> love, just as I have obeyed my Father's commands and remain
> in his love.
> (John 15:9–10)

The relationship of family is characterized by love and is a safe
and secure place to be. The joy and intimacy of having God
as Father is also reflected in the way Jesus prays to him using
the word *Abba*, encouraging us to use this term to talk to him
as our Father too.

Jesus calls us brothers (and sisters!)

This family includes not only other sinful human beings like
ourselves, but also Jesus himself. God is our Father and Jesus
is pleased to be our Brother:

Both the one who makes men holy and those who are made holy are of the same family. So Jesus is not ashamed to call them brothers. He says,

'I will declare your name to my brothers;
  in the presence of the congregation I will sing
    your praises.'
(Hebrews 2:11–12)

Jesus wants to praise God with us! We do not know that as a physical reality now, but it is spiritually true.

The church family

For believers, another spiritual reality is that we have an incredible worldwide Christian family who are here on earth with us, all of whom are our brothers and sisters. This means that we belong, that we can be loved and cherished. We have responsibilities for one another. We are to be loyal and sacrificial, and we are to nurture one another. Yes, I definitely do have a family! This is how David described the reality of facing infertility within the church family:

We know that many are praying for us and want to love and support us through it. Once in a while someone will say something really helpful that will move us to tears. The love of God's people is a wonderful thing.

There will of course be many times when our church family lets us down. Our earthly Christian family will not always get it right. That is why Jesus taught us that we need to put him first.

Christ first

In Mark 3:34–35, Jesus famously put the family of believers before his own biological family. 'Then he looked at those seated in a circle around him and said, "Here are my mother and my brothers! Whoever does God's will is my brother and sister and mother."' Here he stressed that our family allegiance to God is even stronger than our allegiance to a physical family. Jesus had understood this back at the age of twelve when he went missing from Mary and Joseph on the way back from Jerusalem. He considers his place in Joseph's *bêt 'āb* as less significant than his position as God's Son when he refers to the temple as 'my Father's house' (Luke 2:49).

The idea that devotion to God is more precious than anything else, even family, is an extraordinary claim to make in today's society. Even so, we cannot neglect our responsibilities towards parents and siblings while we serve God.

Who am I if I do not have a family of my own?

In the course of talking to women and giving seminars on this topic, we have heard many articulate a frustration that they do not feel they are living out what they were made for in their other family – the church family. Lizzie and Mary perhaps express this most clearly:

Lizzie
Well, I know I am part of God's family in the church, but I'm not clear on the role I should play, given that I have always felt I could serve God best by being a mother. Yet I remain childless. If I can't be a mother, I do not know how to go on.

Mary
*Some of my concerns have been around the issues of role and
purpose, as I have always felt, even before marriage, that I had strong
maternal feelings and qualities, and I struggle to understand how to
deal with these in facing childlessness.*

Mary and Lizzie's description of their struggle for identity
poses questions that dig deep into aspects of the core identity of all of us, whether single or married, male or female.
Who am I? What is my role? What value do I have? How is
our identity shaped by being part of God's spiritual family,
whether we are single or married? I (Sue) clearly identify
with Mary's strong maternal feelings. I felt that I had a vast
untapped and unused resource in me for loving and caring for
children. I longed to use those qualities and I thought it was
such a waste not to be able to do so. As Kimberly Monroe puts
it, 'Infertility shatters your identity. You have a picture in your
mind. You are married. You have a house with a white picket
fence. You have a minivan and a big dog. But where are the
children?'[2]

So, in trying to address some of these issues, it might be
useful to start by examining what or who defines my identity.

Made in the image of a Father God

Genesis 1:27 tells us that we are made in the image of God.

> So God created man
>   in his own image,
> in the image of God
>   he created him;
> male and female
>   he created them.

The description of God's love for Israel described in Hosea 11:1–4 gives us an insight into what God is like: 'When Israel was a child, I loved him, and out of Egypt I called my son.' This is the God in whose image we are made: a God who loves as a perfect Father, a kind, compassionate, patient, loving Father. We are made with the 'stamp' or 'mark' of a parent. So it is a very natural part of our identity to love and nurture others. No wonder then that we find infertility and childlessness hard.

It may seem counterproductive to make us in this image and then deny our ability to be a parent. However, that could assume that 'parenting' is worked out only with our own offspring. It may be surprising to see that parenting qualities are not used in the New Testament to encourage people to be better parents to their children. Of course, a natural outworking of these attributes is with one's own children. But in the New Testament it's interesting to note who has the skills that one might attribute *only* to mums and dads.

Parental love in the church

The New Testament is awash with the analogy of parents' love for their children when describing the conduct, role, attitude and love that Paul has for Christians – Paul, a single man! In his letters, Paul states time and time again that the way he loves his fellow Christians is as a father loves his children. He uses the analogy of a loving parent to plead with them, encourage and rebuke them. So in 1 Corinthians 4:14 he protectively warns them: 'I am not writing this to shame you, but to warn you, as my dear children.' In 2 Corinthians 6:11–13 he intimately pleads with the Corinthians to open their hearts to him:

> We have spoken freely to you, Corinthians, and opened
> wide our hearts to you. We are not withholding our affection
> from you, but you are withholding yours from us. As a fair
> exchange – I speak as to my children – open wide your hearts
> also.

And in Galatians 4:19–20 he uses the extraordinary analogy of giving birth to describe his toil and service for these Christians: 'My dear children, for whom I am again in the pains of childbirth until Christ is formed in you, how I wish I could be with you now and change my tone, because I am perplexed about you!'

Paul reminds the Thessalonians of his love for them, expressed in gentleness as he 'mothered' and 'fathered' them:

> As apostles of Christ we could have been a burden to you,
> but we were gentle among you, like a mother caring for her
> little children. We loved you so much that we were delighted
> to share with you not only the gospel of God but our lives
> as well, because you had become so dear to us . . .
>
>   For you know that we dealt with each of you as a father
> deals with his own children, encouraging, comforting and
> urging you to live lives worthy of God, who calls you into his
> kingdom and glory.
> (1 Thessalonians 2:6b–8, 11–12)

And there's more! Paul calls Timothy and Titus his 'true son(s) in the faith' (1 Timothy 1:2; Titus 1:4). 1 John is written to 'my dear children' (1 John 2:1). And all this is modelled on Jesus' love for his disciples; he calls his disciples 'My children' (John 13:33).

The emotive and intimate language of parental love is primarily used to illustrate the love, care and concern that single men (Jesus, Paul, John) had for other adults growing up as Christians within the spiritual family – which begs the question, 'Why do we have this model?'

Parenting qualities principally benefit the church

As Christians, we are made in the image of a loving parent so that we can use these 'parenting skills' in a much wider sense than with just our own children: to love, nurture and care for our fellow Christians. For the sake of building up his church, God has given us *this* identity, the identity of a loving mother/father.

This identity is in all of us, whether we have children or not, whether we are single or married. For those who are married, this radical identity of being 'parents' to other Christians is there whether you have children or not. So, when two become one, a new family unit is created: a family unit that exists with or without children. For those who are single, an identity of a loving father/mother can be embraced alone, knowing that in God's economy as part of his body, the church, you have all you need to 'parent' other Christians.

It's as if the *prime reason* for these 'parenting skills' is to equip us to love and care for our fellow Christians. John himself says that nothing could be more important: 'I have no greater joy than to hear that my children are walking in the truth' (3 John 4).

This is how Belinda put it:

> I do believe that a man and his wife constitute the family; as the biblical 'one flesh', we are already a family unit and the Lord brings us people to care for into that unit, whether or not they are our own flesh and blood.

I don't feel very maternal/paternal

Some Christian couples have admitted struggling to deal with an absence of maternal or paternal feelings. This is Fiona's struggle in this area:

> I'm not the sort of person who naturally warms towards children or who wants to pick up and cuddle a baby. I don't have confidence that I could love a child well. I am anxious about children and feel a guilty relief that I haven't had any. It's not acceptable to be reluctant to be a mother. I'm ashamed of my struggle, and most conversations assume that I want a child desperately.

The obvious reply was, 'Once you have your own child you'll feel differently.' For many people who subsequently have children, those parental feelings inevitably do materialize. There may be many different reasons for reluctance or anxiety about being a parent, such as one's expectations about the feelings/nature one should have, difficulties in marriage, fears from childhood patterns, lack of confidence or distrust of one's own character. It is important to talk about this together as a couple and to someone else you can both trust. Paul David Tripp in his book *Lost in the Middle* writes about being able to face up to the exposure of one's inabilities and not being paralysed by them, because of God's amazing grace. I cannot commend this book highly enough, for though it deals with midlife, the issues and struggles described apply to all of us who are struggling with identity in some measure.

But struggles such as Fiona's can freeze us in the present, especially when this reluctance or absence of desire becomes a reason to avoid pursuing fertility investigations or treatment. Coping with this ongoing guilt in the event of subsequent infertility is wearing. Conversations with professional counsellors might provide some very useful insights into the reasons for an absence of maternal/paternal feelings. And it may be that repentance is needed in some areas, as understanding and insights come to light. But perhaps the focus could be shifted, so that, in the face of ongoing infertility, instead of trying to whip up maternal/paternal feelings for children who have not been given to you, you could seek to invest your God-given parental qualities in those around you in your church family. How can you seek to love, care, support and nurture those people now?

7 The expectations of others

Trudy

Infertility is a lonely and chronic grief. I found that people didn't understand – it was not as if you'd actually had something and lost it, so why the grief? It was too painful and personal to share with people at our Bible study group, so I said nothing.

Kath

Few people in the church and among friends or family understand or even remember that this is such a problem for me/us. Even if they remember, they forget to ask or are too embarrassed to do so. Most of the time I am screaming inwardly for people to ask me how I am, to give me a cuddle, or simply to listen and not say anything.

Trudy and Kath's experiences show that, even though the church is in theory the place where those struggling with infertility should feel supported and loved, many find attending church is hard for different reasons. The ever-present children are a constant reminder of what they don't have. Time and again women have said that there was no-one they felt they could go to for support. Often they are on the receiving end of clumsy questions, which are poorly thought through, exposing raw wounds. It's difficult to know how to reveal our experience of infertility when it is never mentioned publicly in church. We don't know how much we should talk about it to others, without causing embarrassment at our grief. It's so hard to be positive when someone else's pregnancy is announced. Words elude us to articulate the struggle that no-one appears to be aware of.

Going to church is so hard

Lorna and Andy
We found going to church painful sometimes, surrounded by many young families who seemed to produce children effortlessly. We recall battling with jealousy.

The danger is that Trudy, Kath, Lorna and Andy all might stop going to church if they find it too painful.

The writer to the Hebrews deals with exactly this temptation:

> And let us consider how we may spur one another on
> towards love and good deeds. Let us not give up meeting
> together, as some are in the habit of doing, but let us
> encourage one another – and all the more as you see the
> Day approaching.
> (Hebrews 10:24–25)

So Trudy and Kath need to be encouraged to keep going to church, not only so that they can be prayed for, but also so they can pray for and encourage others.

Susannah penned her struggle in response to these verses:

At times I used to dread going to church, simply because I would be surrounded by healthy fertile women and bouncing babies. Everyone was getting pregnant at the drop of a hat. In my self-centredness (at times) and pain, I couldn't see that it was precisely my church family who were best equipped to help me in my struggle. I needed clear teaching to remind me about the hope of heaven. I needed to be reminded that although my journey with infertility was painful, I had a map to guide me continually and keep me on the right path. The map was the Word of God to teach, rebuke, correct and train me in righteousness. But I also needed Christian friends to remind me they were praying for me, and I needed to hear of others' struggles to put mine in perspective.

So Christian men and women who find attending church difficult because of the presence of many children need encouragement to help them keep going as they serve their church family.

Other people's questions and comments

Tom

Often people ask, 'Do you have children?' I once caught myself answering this question from a work colleague with 'We tried, but it didn't happen for us', when I realized that that was not what she was asking, but whether I wanted the toy from her Big Mac Happy Meal! A look of 'too much information' swept across her face. But it is sometimes difficult to gauge what is appropriate when asked such seemingly banal questions. I work on a children's ward and I have been asked many times, 'Do you have children?' to which I am compelled to say, 'No', which translates to them as 'You have no understanding of our suffering then.' In fact I was castigated once,

'Well, when you choose to have children, you might understand how we feel.' It is the presumption of choice that sticks in the throat.

Peter and Vivienne
The reality of the loss of fertility set in hard, particularly as friends began to announce pregnancies and celebrate new births, often with little tact. It seemed that people expected more from us, rather than empathizing with our situation as we confronted a very difficult but 'invisible' problem. A few close friends were, and have continued to be, faithfully supportive, but others withdrew as the months passed, and we also received our share of wrong-headed 'counsel': for example, in effect, 'You haven't lost anything'; 'God doesn't want you to have children'; or 'Stop being miserable and be happy for others.'

Mary
It was important to us that people weren't over-fussy with sympathy, trying to hard to make everything better.

You will come across a whole range of comments from the mean, the clumsy to the over-the-top supportive. Some people will say things because they feel awkward or embarrassed. Others will want to try to 'rescue' you from your sadness by offering some kind of hope.

As someone on the receiving end of some of these comments, I (Sue) have often gritted my teeth inwardly and struggled not to make a tart response. How you react will vary according to your relationship with that person and how you are coping at the time. At times it will be legitimate to say nothing, absorb the hurt, accept others' failings graciously and not bear a grudge. At other times, it may be worth a gentle challenge at an appropriate time, so as to avoid someone else being hurt by a repetition of those same comments. The challenge could be about the timing/place/lack of insight, or about the biblical basis for the comment. But it's also important not be so uptight about others' comments that you end up having people walking on eggshells around you for fear of unwittingly upsetting you.

How about that question, 'Do you have children?' It might be worth developing a stock answer which helps the questioner, rather than focusing on you, and which points to gratitude to God for what he has done rather than what he hasn't. Something like, 'No, we don't and, although we would love to have had children, we know that God has not forgotten us and has graciously provided.' This speaks of your trust in God and helps keep you thankful in him.

When a pregnancy is announced

Hope
On occasion, I am bitter towards those who have multiple children.
I cannot stand people who moan about what hard work kids are.
The thing guaranteed to send me running from a room is to hear a
story of 'falling' pregnant unplanned.

Pregnancies will be hard to hear of, more so at some times than others, depending on how close you are to the one announcing the pregnancy. The tenderness and grief when struggling with infertility is so raw at times, that hearing the news of another's pregnancy can rip open wounds and cause fresh hurt. This is often compounded by guilt at not feeling happy for the other person. Many women find this an ongoing struggle. And sometimes it doesn't get any easier. As someone who has been dealing with infertility for seventeen years, I (Sue) need to be careful that I don't create such an aura of protectiveness around myself that people are afraid to share this good news with me.

It is something to commit to prayer, as a new life is always a good thing for the whole community to rejoice over. The practical outworking of what genuine love in the church looks like in Romans 12:15 covers the Christian's response to both sets of circumstances of good and bad news: 'Rejoice with those who rejoice; mourn with those who mourn.'

To go on loving, when you're aching with sadness inside, is such a challenge. I (Sue) found it really helpful to remember that the fullest description of love in the New Testament in 1 Corinthians 13 does not have anything to do with feelings. The figure of speech used to describe love is principally verbs, or as we learnt at school, 'doing' words. Waiting for the feeling before you do or say something loving is often a guarantee that you won't ever do anything! However wooden you may sound, saying, 'It's great that you are pregnant, thanks to God' conveys love to the other. This is not being hypocritical. It is part of the Christian discipline of not letting relationships be governed purely by your internal state.

I can't cope with Mother's Day

Mary
Particular church events continue to be challenging, and I have chosen to avoid over-exposure to child-related events at present.

Mother's Day can be routinely avoided by people struggling with infertility. I (Sue) remember being in tears as flowers were handed out by all the children to their mums. For those who lead church services, it might be helpful to think through how Mother's Day can be sensitively celebrated in a church situation where many single and married women will be automatically left on the sidelines.

The choice not to attend services like this may be initially entirely legitimate and serve as self-protection. Of course this may not just be the case for those struggling with childlessness. But for those who find this day hard and choose not to go, be prepared to rethink this over the years and to pray for an ease of the pain to make this day more bearable and to consider participating. This is not meant to sound harsh, but gently to challenge those 'fixed' positions we may adopt as we grieve – the no-go areas.

8 Keeping marriage strong

Trudy

It's painful for me to look back over those early years of our marriage. We already had problems, particularly in dealing with conflict. I'd brought rather a lot of childhood angst to our marriage, and the added burden of infertility was almost too much to bear. I felt an all-round failure as a wife and as a woman.

Fiona

Our experience on getting married was that alongside finding communication, leadership and submission difficult, we found making love difficult. Our response to this over time was to distance ourselves from each other and 'abandon the project' as far as sex was concerned. We thought we might as well just get along without it, that sex was optional in marriage. I was disappointed and confused as to what the point of sex was. We didn't talk about having children, but that was all bound up with sex, and we'd found that didn't work for us. We didn't talk about that either. Our relationship became more distant. Our conviction is that marriage is for life, so divorce wasn't an option. Neither of us considered it. We just settled for two rather independent lives, more like colleagues or siblings than husband and wife.

Marriages dealing with infertility, like Trudy's and Fiona's, can come under a huge strain, whether this is through the distractions of assisted conception, adoption or simply accepting childlessness. This may lead to misunderstandings, poor communication and grievances that can take years to resolve. And these are compounded by the husband and wife potentially grieving very differently, to varying degrees, and at separate times.

Some couples may not be able to talk about their grief with each other. Sex may be an area of disharmony, disappointment, tension and dissatisfaction. Trying to maintain a healthy marriage is a real challenge.

Consider your expectations

Tom

I think my wife felt she had let me down by not providing a son to carry on the family name and so on, but I think the significance of this issue was much greater in her mind than it ever was in mine.

Expectations cover all sorts of areas, not only about children, but also about daily living patterns, social arrangements, recreation, church money, work, housing, sex, spiritual ministry and family. Often these expectations aren't articulated, yet they do exist. They are formed by a whole host of experiences as a child or an adult.

We all had and have expectations of our spouses and marriage. Expectations aren't necessarily right or wrong, but if left unidentified and unexamined, they can pave the way for misunderstanding, poor communication and disappointment between couples. Friction in marriage, or in any relationship, can often arise from people having differing expectations and assumptions.

In his excellent book *Married for God* Christopher Ash's stated intention at the outset is to consider 'What ought our purpose to be? What are proper hopes and aims for marriages?'[1] At the end of each chapter he poses questions that help to identify expectations in many different areas of marriage. It is an extremely helpful resource for engaged or married couples, which could also be used by individuals for self-reflection.

Develop a healthy sex life

God created sex to be good. The sexual delights of pleasure, deep intimacy and orgasm are designed by God. But alongside this we live in a fallen world, where such experiences may often be marred by the complexities of the fall and our sinfulness. Sex can easily become an idol, even within marriage. So sex is good, but sex is fallen.

Childlessness is renowned for turning lovemaking into a chore. It may seem a long time since we heard these words at our own marriage: 'Marriage is given . . . that with delight and tenderness they may know each other in love, and, through the joy of their bodily union, may strengthen the union of their hearts and lives.'[2] The joy of bodily union can become lost amid choosing the best time of the month and optimal body positioning! Our motives are entirely caught up with the potential conception, rather than focusing on each other and giving each other pleasure. At the 'wrong' times of the month, lovemaking can be left to one side as an unappealing reminder of the situation. For those going through fertility treatment, sex may cease to be an intimate union between husband and wife. There may be guilt at not enjoying sex any more. What was once private is now 'owned' by a medical team.

Physical difficulties, such as impotence, erectile dysfunction, vaginal discomfort and other medical conditions, will all have physical and psychological bearings on your sexual relationship. And if any of these make lovemaking near impossible, there are the additional potential responses of guilt and anger if conception is never given a chance.

Fiona

My husband and I have struggled with sex right from the beginning . . . it feels so very shameful to admit sexual failure. The marriage preparation course we attended never broached the subject of difficulty with sex. We didn't know that it could be difficult and didn't know what to do if it was . . . My biggest problem right now is my marriage, not my childlessness.

A sexual relationship is affected by tension, disappointment and sadness. Gender differences may be apparent – women may find it harder to enjoy spontaneous sex outside 'planned' times, men may become deeply dissatisfied by the lack of spontaneity. There will be exceptions to this of course, but the question will inevitably arise: 'What is the point of sex?' What is its overall purpose in marriage?

Paul reminds us of God's will for us to keep sex alive within marriage – not for the sake of making babies, but with the aim of gluing two people together in their hearts and in their lives:

The husband should fulfil his marital duty to his wife, and likewise the wife to her husband. The wife's body does not belong to her alone but also to her husband. In the same way, the husband's body does not belong to him alone but also to his wife. Do not deprive each other except by mutual consent and for a time, so that you may devote yourselves to prayer.

> Then come together again so that Satan will not tempt you
> because of your lack of self-control.
> (1 Corinthians 7:3–5)

Even though sex is fallen, it is still good. In fact in marriage,
sex is crucial – so crucial that Paul strongly advises against
abstinence in marriage in 1 Corinthians 7:5. He recognizes the
temptation caused by a lack of self-control. In other words, if
you deprive each other of sex in marriage ('except by mutual
consent and for a time'), you are putting each other at risk of
being sexually tempted by someone else. So sex is never an
end in itself.

Making love has a powerful role in keeping husband and
wife faithful to each other. Paul never mentions procreation
in 1 Corinthians 7 in his justification for frequent marital sex.
But in case we use this to justify a self-indulgent obsession
with inward-looking intimacy alone, we need reminding
of the 'joint stewarding' task given to Adam and Eve. Guy
Brandon acknowledges that 'the church has often neglected
the wider task of stewarding, or failed to set procreation
within an appropriate framework, and so placed too much
emphasis on childbearing – which causes confusion or stress
for couples who cannot have children'.[3] He helpfully clarifies
this broader remit of 'the job-related, outward-looking task
of stewarding creation which includes cultural and social as
well as economic responsibilities'. So, in childless marriages,
we can take comfort in the fact that there are very important
reasons for the husband and wife to continue offering their
bodies to each other.

Your sexual relationship is another area of 'expectations'.
Have you and your spouse talked about how often each of
you would like to, or expected to, make love? What helps to
'set the scene' sexually? What gets you sexually excited in each

other? Couples will differ in how much they talk about sex and what vocabulary they use. But if you never talk about sex or your own sexual needs, there is a risk you may make the wrong assumptions, leaving one partner feeling sexually unsatisfied. This could lead to bitterness, lack of forgiveness, and grief within a marriage.

It may be worth thinking through what has informed your ideas of sex and seeing how this impacts on your expectations. Our culture tells us lies about sex. As Lauren Winner puts it, 'Our popular culture has turned sex into a bulwark against and a refuge from the commonplace and ordinary practices of marriage. It has created a falsely romantic ideal of sexual love.'[4]

It is generally unhelpful to judge the quality of your marriage by the frequency or quality of lovemaking. Bear in mind 1 Corinthians 7, that it is more important to have sex (even if it's not 'great' sex) than not to have any. Both husbands and wives need to take responsibility for heeding this command to go on having sex even when it is really difficult. A husband needs to make this area of the marriage a priority, persevering despite embarrassment, even when he may need to ask for help. Paul tells us that if he doesn't, Satan will make the most of the situation, usually by distracting the man's attention elsewhere. The devil may tempt through the attractions of recreational sex, or he may remind husbands more frequently and more insistently of sexual temptation on the Internet. This threat is real. Denying one another sexually can lead to a lack of trust and insecurity in every area of the marriage.

Marital sex should do far more than provide personal pleasure and a better quality of relationship. Within marriage, sex cultivates faithfulness, service and loving fruitfulness. As Christopher Ash puts it:

Sex must be put in its proper place in marriage. On the one hand, it is not the be-all and end-all of marriage. Sex is not a god or goddess; sex cannot save us or give us our identity or fulfilment. But, on the other hand, sex is very important and the sexual relationship needs to be nurtured as the heart of a relationship of faithful love . . . So we must nurture sex, but not as an end in itself. We nurture the private intimacy of marriage in order to keep fires burning that will warm others outside.[5]

Serving in the church and beyond

Our marriages can also be strengthened through testing times by focusing on the ways in which we can serve our church family together.

David
I am a pastor in a church and I am used to carrying the burdens of others. I am aware of those in the church who are also struggling with infertility. I am also aware of a number of single women who can hear the clock ticking and who want to be married and have children before it's too late. For that reason my wife and I have decided to be as open as possible about our infertility. And we've found that very helpful.

The situation of being without children may bring surprising opportunities. It may not diminish the sadness or the heartache, but it may bring a new perspective to what is happening. We are called to serve with the gifts that God has given us and, in facing childlessness, God is training us in unique ways that will help to build up the body of Christ.

Just as each of us has one body with many members, and these members do not all have the same function, so in Christ we who are many form one body, and each member belongs to all the others. We have different gifts according to the grace given us.

(Romans 12:4–6a)

What gifts does God give us through our experiences of childlessness?

Empathy: The most obvious benefit to the church is the gift of understanding that we have been given. Even if we go on to have children, we know exactly what it is like to have been in this position. To develop this gift, it is useful to have kept a journal during the difficult times, so that we are able to go back and remember the heartache. This is not so that we will say, 'I know what that feels like', since people respond to infertility in different ways. It just makes us more patient as we listen and more ready to grieve with those who grieve.

Prayer: If we have been driven to our knees by an experience that we have no control over, we will be more ready to urge our friends to pray too. We will know that entrusting our fears and struggles to the Lord is a vital part of living without the children that we long for. We will also want to pray more on our own and will probably support the church prayer meeting more readily.

Resources: The simple fact is that without children you will have more time to do the things that you would like to do. Now the struggle is between you and your willpower to put the right proportion of that time to work in serving the church. There will be more money around without the costs of bringing up children! Where will this money go instead? Will the wider church benefit?

William

As time went by, we naturally became more accepting of our situation and enjoyed other people's children, either in the family or with friends, and we also realized that the very fact that we did not have the 'tie' of children meant that we were able to do things together which would not have been possible if we had family responsibilities. Linda was able to join me on my business travels, for example. She was certainly given an important and effective ministry with the women of our church, running Bible studies and other activities for many years with a degree of commitment and involvement that would have been impossible for a mother with children to care for.

The challenges to use our gifts are the same for everyone, no matter what types of trials we are facing. Are we able to look up and look around at the needs around us? If all things are working for the good of those who love God, how can our painful experiences work to build others up?

9 Real men experience infertility

William

Men can be very cruel. I will never forget a Christian friend bursting into the office to announce, 'I am a man!' It was his way of telling us that he was going to be a father. The inference was obvious and, although in my better moments I can dismiss it, I have never forgotten it or how inadequate it made me feel at the time! Even so, I think that this period was most difficult for Linda, but my struggles seemed to come later, as I would see my contemporaries taking their children swimming or dancing or to watch or play football or cricket. This bonding of a father with his son or daughter is something I would long to experience, and I knew I never would.

Anyone knows that to be a real man you do not have to have children. You don't even need to be married. But in the context of office or locker-room banter, it seems that the opposite is true. When William's friend declared himself 'a man' because he had managed to fertilize an egg, he was way off in his understanding, but the coarse jokes and comments that men may overhear can cause fear and resentment for life.

In the Bible, when a man is created, the emphasis is on the fact that he is made in God's image. He takes responsibility for the animals and for the earth. Yet the area of his life that is most important is his relationship with God. He is to listen to God's Word and obey it. This is the emphasis that we see in the life of Jesus. Despite all the pressures that he faces, his main concern is to look to his Father God for guidance and strength. This was the case in the desert when he was tempted by the devil to turn the stones into bread. He answered, 'It is written: "Man does not live on bread alone, but on every word that comes from the mouth of God"' (Matthew 4:4). We are encouraged to put our relationship with God and obedience to his Word at the centre of everything, particularly when times are tough.

Trevor found out recently that his latest investigative operation had retrieved no mature sperm whatsoever. Stacey simultaneously went through an IVF (*in vitro* fertilization) cycle to harvest her eggs to be ready for fertilization just in case his results were positive, but in the event there was nothing to add to them. For this couple, it was the conclusive end to a two-year journey of tests and operations to find some way to have a baby.

Trevor has kept a journal for much of this time and has thought a great deal about the issues that men face in the light of infertility, especially when a lack of sperm is the main problem. He writes here about three particular issues that he has identified as significant for men:

Identity

My feelings about identity kicked off after I had my testicle removed over four years ago, even though I didn't know at that point that I'd never be able to father a child. When I received the results of the sperm test, it was a huge shock; my view of myself was turned

completely upside down. Maybe it was because of the view that I'd
had as a young man coming out of university, fairly sporty, ready
to take on the world, that I experienced this massive flip in identity.
I could only think, Wow, where does that leave me in terms of
who I am as a bloke?

It's not that I don't know the answer – that my identity is rooted
in being a child of God. I know that, but it is still a constant battle.
I keep on feeling fearful and unconfident and 'less male' because of
my infertility. It is one of those Christian battles that I will always
have to fight. A year ago I caved in. I had what felt like an early
onset of midlife crisis between January and March, and the whole
thing overwhelmed me. Who was I? What was I doing? What
was my meaning, my purpose? I felt very flat and wanted to break
out. I even wanted to buy a sports car! I would go to work and think,
I don't want to be here. Yet I would spend all of my energy at work,
trying to find meaning and value there. When I came home my
energy was all used up and I would lie uselessly on the sofa being
completely uncommunicative to Stacey.

One of the things that we've often talked of as a couple is the fact
that Jesus is the most manly example of a guy, and he didn't have any
children. I read a book called Men: Firing Through All of Life by
Al Stewart. It helped me to understand that male identity has got to be
tied up with our adoption as children and being part of God's family.
Whether or not you have children, you are part of God's family. This
gave us real strength.

Within my own family background, we were brought up to be
aware of the certainty of God's unconditional love for each of us,
and my parents sought to reflect that as a principle. However, I have
a very strong Christian father as a role model, and my perception
of his expectations created difficulties for me in terms of my own
identity. He is very caring and is trying to encourage us as we go
through this, but he has seemingly found it difficult to demonstrate
his own emotions. This has made me feel that being manly is about

not being upset – it's about keeping a stiff upper lip! Perhaps this is just his personality, but even so, I wish that he would talk to me about how he felt, tell me that it was a hard situation and that it was difficult to deal with, especially when my parents had said that they had had their own problems conceiving. I wish that he had validated the way that I felt and told me that it was all right to be upset and that there were no easy answers.

The one thing that has really kept us going is knowing that God is our perfect Father and that God understands the way we feel even when we are incapable of understanding it ourselves. That is still the case even if we're not the biological father of a child. We're fathered by a Father who hears and understands us, and who wants to help us.

Coping with friends, relatives and colleagues

It seems to me that we need to ask, 'What does it look like to be dealing well with the situation I find myself in?' 'What is a godly way to cope with tragedy?' I found in my crisis that I was expected to cope. I reacted by putting a mask on so that it looked as though I was doing exactly that. I tried to show that I was keeping all of the balls up in the air at the same time. I really think that men need to be told that it's okay to sit down and bawl their eyes out for three hours. It's okay not to cope. Not to do anything. Just to stop and cry.

I told my boss at work about what was happening and he told me to take a week off. I didn't and I regret that now. Someone else would have had to take my workload on and, because it was at a time when very few colleagues were aware of what was happening, I knew that people would be questioning why I wasn't there. I thought, look, we're Christians here in this place, and if we're falling apart at the merest sign of crisis, then people are going to feel that Christianity doesn't hold up. It is a ridiculous view but it does go through your mind. You read about all these Christians who

*present amazing witnesses of holding up under terrible suffering
and showing how amazing the gospel is, and you want to be like
that. Your pride feels dented when you are unable to be like that
and it hurts. What you do and who you are has been blown out of
the water by the terrible news, and you try to pick yourself up by
doing other things well.*

*When we first started telling people about eighteen months ago,
they would mostly say, 'Oh well, I'm sure there is something that
they can do.' The most intelligent comment actually came from my
line manager who turned around and said, 'That's complete rubbish,
isn't it', with slightly stronger words! It was a relief to hear him say
that and one of the most helpful comments I've had, because it was
recognizing that this was all really tough.*

Relating to wives

*My natural instinct was to go into 'protector mode'. I felt that I had
to provide theological answers to solve the situation and I expected
that to be enough. I didn't understand why, having given Stacey the
Bible verses, she was still upset! She says that at that time there was
nothing I could have said that would have made any difference, and
all she wanted was for me to hug her and say I loved her. I did do that
sometimes, but the truth is that I simply didn't know how to cope
with her feelings. I thought that I was protecting her by not telling
her what I was going through myself and so adding to her grief. We
were both isolated in our feelings. I became angry and directed my
anger wrongly at Stacey. There was a while when I didn't want to go
home because it was like walking on eggshells, and I was either being
shouted at or had a wife in tears whom I was useless at comforting.
My world was descending into a cycle of madness and chaos that I
was powerless to do anything about. I told her that she would have
been better off marrying someone else. Thankfully, she didn't agree!
When I finally realized that I needed to talk to her, it helped me to get
through some pretty dark times.*

Other men have also made very useful comments about how they have coped and what they have learnt about the best way to look after their wives:

Stephen

Somewhere really early on, I think through reading the Mars and Venus book,[1] I got that message not to try and fix things, which was fortunate, I think. It helps sometimes to be able to say, 'Look, I know this isn't going to fix it, but just let me do a bit of male processing here. I know this isn't a solve-all solution, but as a bloke let me do a bit of hunter-protecting for a moment.' I also found that occasionally (like at a particular time of the month!) it was helpful to throw money at the situation and go and eat somewhere nice or send her off for some clothes shopping.

David

I know that my wife feels an intense longing to have children, but most of the time I do not feel that. I realize that later in my life I probably will. That is not to say that I never feel bad about our childlessness. When I see a young woman with a pushchair, I wish it was my wife. When I sense my wife's heart sinking because she sees the pride on a new mother's face, I grieve for her. When my wife snaps at me because I don't want to make love, I know that behind the snapping is a deep yearning for pregnancy which I want to give her but can't.

David's tender awareness of his wife's struggles brings another dimension to his own struggle. As well as the blow of facing a future without children, men may have to face a future with a wife who has had her dreams shattered. When the man and woman got married, before they started trying for children, 'he' was the answer to all of 'her' hopes and dreams. Before all of this, he was 'simply the best!' Now he may be simply not enough. As Elkanah said to the inconsolable Hannah, 'Hannah, why are you weeping? Why don't you eat? Why are you downhearted? Don't I mean more to you than ten sons?' (1 Samuel 1:8)

Your wife may present you with a whole range of needs, but overall, she needs you to be most concerned for her relationship with the Lord. Throughout the pain and turmoil, somehow you do still need to feed her with God's Word and care for her with the love of Christ. Exactly how you do that in a loving way may be mirrored by Christ's own compassionate attitude for the church: 'Husbands ought to love their wives as their own bodies. He who loves his wife loves himself. After all, no-one ever hated his own body, but he feeds and cares for it, just as Christ does the church' (Ephesians 5:28–29).

Catherine

Luke thought that infertility was a private matter, not for discussion. But for me, talking to my various girlfriends was such a great tonic. I needed to talk and would have found it much harder to get through the process and pain without their support. Those girlfriends that I chose to confide in were incredibly gracious, listening to me for hours on end, which was just so kind and helpful to me.

Catherine's experience is an example of how many women deal with infertility. Although this is a generalization (there are always exceptions), this means that a woman facing infertility will probably find some comfort in talking about it. It may be that she just wants to talk to her husband about it – in which case he needs to be ready, listening and probably not offering those much-feared solutions. She may, however, find that she wants to talk to trusted and caring friends and will need to share private aspects of your situation with them. Consequently some husbands may feel vulnerable and threatened. The husband may need to consider how he could anticipate his wife's needs.

It's not a guy thing, but even so, ask for help when you need it

As Trevor said earlier, it is okay not to be coping very well and to have fears about the whole issue.

David

I have many fears. I fear that my wife will get pregnant and then lose the baby: I just don't know how I would cope with that. I fear that we will soon get to the point where we start arguing about adoption, which I know we feel differently about. I fear that my wife will be left alone if I die before her.

David's honest fears may leave him paralysed if he doesn't talk about them to someone. It can be a lot less straightforward for a man to talk to his friends about his struggles to have children than it is for a woman. But if he can perhaps go for a drink with a good friend who kind of knows what's up already, then that is a start. Perhaps there is someone a bit older in the church or even someone who has had personal experience of what it is like to face these difficulties. Giving him the opportunity to talk may bring up things that he just needs to hear himself saying.

Nate

I would say that men in general feel very challenged in asking for support. I felt if I told my friends about my infertility and admitted that it is my physical handicap, I would be on the receiving end of

locker-room ridicule and hurtful jokes, even if they were meant as
banter. I guess it would have been worth the risk to reach out to a
man and be blunt and say, 'I just wanted to share this with you
so you know what is going on. You might not have anything to say,
you might not know what to say, but I appreciate you listening and
your prayers, and I don't want this to be weird, but I needed to get
this out.'

A good friend or pastor will want him to know that he can do just that: just to listen and pray. They will also want to gently make sure, when the moment is right, that he is still listening to God's Word and putting it into practice in his life, particularly in his relationship with his wife. They will want him to know how much God cares for him in every detail of his life.

Being a man involves being weak and vulnerable at times, experiencing intense jealousy, rivalry, anger and frustration. It means feeling crushed by disappointment and failure. The strong, mighty and victorious King David was extremely weak at times and was able to articulate his frailty. He said these things:

> Be merciful to me, O Lord, for I am in distress;
>   my eyes grow weak with sorrow,
>   my soul and my body with grief.
> My life is consumed by anguish
>   and my years by groaning;
> my strength fails because of my affliction,
>   and my bones grow weak . . .
> But I trust in you, O Lord;
>   I say, 'You are my God.'
> My times are in your hands.
> (Psalm 31:9–10, 14–15a)

More advice from real men

What other bits of advice can men offer each other to keep themselves sane and their marriages healthy?

Keep it fun: laugh at yourselves as you obey the baby-making rules of sex. Ben Elton wrote the novel *Inconceivable* as a comic take on infertility after his own experience of it all. Watch the film *Maybe Baby*, which may help you to see the frustrations in a different light (be prepared for some strong language, though).

Create some space of your own: it may be going to the gym three times a week or hitting golf balls, but to have a regular time when you are not at work or at home may give you the space you need. Wives will benefit from this too, and may need to encourage men to take time off.

Plan ahead: it has been said that for women, foreplay is about everything that has happened in the previous twenty-four hours leading up to making love, but for men, it is what happens in the previous three minutes!

Carry on articulating to your wife how desirable you find her, especially when she doesn't feel very attractive, particularly when she most wants to be a mother and at times of the day when you are not planning on having sex.

Find some *very* good friends you can share your anecdotes with about the lengths you have been to as you have tried to conceive, friends who are relaxed enough to laugh along with you. These are probably the same friends who will be able to mop you up when things are really bad.

10 Grieving miscarriage, late-term pregnancy loss and secondary infertility

Lorna and Andy

Miscarriages were not in our mind when we conceived and delivered our first child. We conceived again one year later, but ten weeks into the pregnancy, we had a 'missed miscarriage'. Five months later we conceived again. At seven weeks we again were told there was no heartbeat. We were devastated. We prayed for contentment with our one child, not sure that we could face another missed miscarriage. We did go on to conceive again and give birth to our second child. We then suffered a third miscarriage. Three miscarriages we find baffling. Why does the Lord give only to take away?

Hope

The pain of not being able to give our son a brother or sister and have the family we wanted remains a terrible one. A punishment, if I am honest – an affliction.

Susannah

I have never knowingly got pregnant. Realizing now that I am indeed barren and have never conceived makes me feel my grief has no tangible focus. I have nothing to ground it, just a hole of sadness.

Daisy

We had two healthy daughters when our third child was stillborn at thirty weeks' gestation. The grief we felt was in losing a child who we never got the chance to know, in having no memories of her, no knowledge of her character, and yet feeling she was very much part of us, our family.

Each experience of miscarriage, late-term death and infertility brings with it a unique grief to each couple. The pain of each circumstance of childlessness is exclusive to that person, and does not follow 'set' patterns. So it is often difficult to articulate your feelings in a way that makes you feel you are being heard or understood clearly. This may be compounded by a misunderstanding within and between couples.

My wife/husband just doesn't understand how I'm feeling

Within a marriage, couples may grieve differently. Some couples have told how miscarriages drew them together. But others have described a husband and wife mourning their infertility or loss at different times, sometimes perhaps years apart. This can lead to more pain as one partner in marriage struggles to understand the other's perceived 'lack of feelings', as in Ben and Louisa's case:

When you have experienced miscarriage, future miscarriages get a lot harder, unlike a lot of life experiences where you expect to become accustomed to the feelings and slightly numbed by their effect on you. It hurts every time, and it isn't always easy to talk about it with anyone, including your husband.

My grief is harder to bear than yours

As each person's experience of infertility brings its own particular grief, there is a potential for much misunderstanding or presumption by others. There can be a misconception that one person's grief is easier to bear than another's. In an article in the *Sun*, Judy Cogan (in dealing with secondary infertility) identified where the accusatory finger was pointing, and described 'feeling that you should simply be grateful for the child you have when others are still trying for a first'.

Lorna and Andy's pain of three miscarriages caused them to articulate a common question: 'Wouldn't it be better not to conceive than to conceive and lose the baby?' Susannah goes on to write about her childlessness:

> *Sometimes I feel that my pain of infertility is worse than others'. This was brought to light when I read an interview with Bonnie Tyler in* The Times *about her miscarriage. She said she felt that 'it was a blessing in disguise'. Bonnie goes on to talk about the taboo of being barren, that she needed to know she could be pregnant, that she wasn't barren. This made me feel so sad and ashamed, that my childlessness was 'worse' than miscarriage. If my childlessness is taboo, then my sadness is too. Who would understand me?*

There seems to be a misconception – that one circumstance is 'worse' or 'better' than others. But it would be unhelpful and impossible to 'rank' the following list in terms of the degree of suffering caused to men and women: being single and therefore never having the chance of pregnancy; barrenness; one miscarriage; repeated miscarriages; early miscarriages; late miscarriages; stillbirth; miscarriages after conceiving naturally for the first time; miscarriage after fertility treatment; secondary infertility; miscarriage of single children; miscarriage of twins or more.

It is impossible and unhelpful to weigh one's grief up against someone else's. Each person who experiences infertility has to hold up his or her particular struggle to the description and examples of suffering in the Bible and to an understanding of God and his character, if we are to help one another grieve in a godly way. Unfortunately the Bible doesn't contain all the specific examples of infertility. But there are general principles we can bring to bear.

It's okay to mourn

Crying out to God about what you have lost, or what you don't have, whatever your circumstances, does not mean that you are being unfaithful. Jesus mourned over the death of Lazarus. Job, described as blameless and upright, one who feared God and turned away from evil, mourned his great losses. And God does respond as you turn to him.

God knows your grief

Tom
It struck me that with a stillbirth you at least have a grave and you have a grief that others can see and share in, but with childlessness you don't even have that – it is to grieve all alone.

To the charge that God seems to hide himself in times of trouble, the Psalms comfort us that God hears our cry: 'You hear, O LORD, the desire of the afflicted; you encourage them, and you listen to their cry' (Psalm 10:17). Although our grief feels invisible to all but ourselves, we can be assured that God sees each tear:

You keep track of all my sorrows.

> You have collected all my tears in your bottle.

> You have recorded each one in your book.

(Psalm 56:8)[1]

Psalm 34:18 tells us that this is precisely when God comes alongside and provides comfort, namely when you are feeling grief-stricken: 'The LORD is close to the broken-hearted and saves those who are crushed in spirit.'

Godly grief cries out to God, reminding him of his character and promises to meet us in our grief and to draw near to those who are saddened. We can cling to God's holiness to keep us from falling, and because he is holy, he *himself* is able to keep us from falling.[2]

Focusing on God

Daisy wrote this some time after her third daughter was stillborn:

> We learnt about the object of our trust. Was it in being able to discern reasons why the Lord allowed [her] to die; was it in the 'good' we might see accomplished because of her death? We learnt that all faith is misplaced unless its object is the character of God himself, not circumstances, not outcomes or reasons. For a while I found it easier to believe in God as my Judge, rather than as a loving, generous, gracious Father. I remember my husband challenging me to hold both aspects of God's character together, that he hadn't stopped being loving, good and kind just because our daughter had died.

Annie and Jack have opted to forgo fertility treatment. They put it like this:

We accept that life isn't always about having everything you wish for. In today's society, this is a difficult concept to take on board. However, when you do realize this and leave your life in God's hand, a trust sets in so that, when things don't go right, you always have the knowledge that he is there to help you.

These responses show us that godly comfort can come from placing your trust in God's character alone as he ordains life and death.

God is sovereign over life

When grief is raw and palpable, it's hard to keep the perspective that God is sovereign. Psalm 139 assures us that God knew each of us, even before our bodies were formed. Not only that, but before we had life, God knew how long each of us would live:

> My frame was not hidden from you
>> when I was made in the secret place.
> When I was woven together in the depths of the earth,
>> your eyes saw my unformed body.
> All the days ordained for me
>> were written in your book
>> before one of them came to be.
> (Psalm 139:15–16)

After suffering three miscarriages, Lorna and Andy say:

We know that Job was right in saying that the Lord gives and the Lord takes away. Job assures us that there is such a thing as innocent suffering in God's world. We believe God is sovereign, so we trust that we will meet our unborn children in heaven.

At the funeral of his stillborn daughter, Sam wrote of the pastor's talk from 2 Samuel 12:23b (David's reaction to the news of the death of his and Bathsheba's child): 'I will go to him, but he will not return to me.'

I still find this verse a great help on many levels, not least because of the value given to one child in a world where thousands perish every hour, and particularly a child conceived following David and Bathsheba's adultery. This reminder of God's mercy and grace expressed in David's prayer for the life of his child was, and remains, a source of assurance. At the time I also took the sentence to mean more than that one day David too would die. 'I will go to him . . . ' spoke to me of the hope of reunion in the kingdom of God.

Our hope and sure knowledge is that God alone knows the child who has been miscarried. He has formed this life. He alone knows his or her character, hair colour, personality. And he holds the memory of this little one's precious short-lived life.

Christians who suffer also wait

Mary
The time of waiting has sometimes felt like a void, and very directionless. I have learnt to trust in God but am perhaps still dwelling on the things he hasn't done rather than all the things he has done for us.

Hope was unable to conceive again after her son was born:

I want to be able to leave it there and say, 'That's my story – thank you, God', but I'm not there yet.

Christians struggling with various aspects of childlessness and infertility often express that they feel in a kind of limbo. Hope and Mary's struggle to come to terms with what has happened to them is an ongoing one. We know that one day when the Lord returns we will see clearly, but we question how we should respond to God now as we wait for that day.

Philip Monroe picks up this theme of waiting, in an article written specifically about the pain of infertility: 'Christians who suffer also wait. This is not the passive waiting of stoic endurance. It is an active resting in the goodness of God . . . Godly waiting meditates on God's character, requires self-examination [and] safeguards our hearts.'[3] This often takes time, and requires a commitment to depend on God's character of faithfulness and trustworthiness as you struggle to understand his purposes. Philip Monroe goes on to write that this waiting is not necessarily 'peaceful'; it involves crying out to God to deliver us and show us where we need to change to become more like him.

Reflecting on chapters 6 – 10

Something to read

Bible passages that have been recommended by some of our contributors: Lamentations 3; Psalm 34; Psalm 116; James 1:1–4.

How do the writers of these books encourage Christians to respond to affliction? How would the writer of Lamentations have us 'wait' for the Lord?

Something to do

As a couple, find time to do things together which build up your relationship and which are fun.

A conversation to have

Talk to your pastor about how much emphasis is put on announcing spiritual births in the church alongside physical ones.

For friends and pastors

It's helpful if the news of someone else's pregnancy is broken quite early on, so that the person struggling with infertility doesn't hear it through the grapevine. It's also helpful to think of how the news will be received, and how support and love can be shown when this news will be hard to take.

Marriage preparation classes: Do you teach the whole truth about sex in marriage preparation classes? Do you teach that sex is sometimes difficult, painful or frustrating? Consider adding the possibility of infertility to the topics you cover. How can you encourage couples to think about how they might react if one or both were diagnosed with a fertility problem?

Don't assume wives and husbands are supporting each other. It may be worth asking a question such as, 'Are you able to talk about this with your husband / wife?', or more directly, 'Where do you get support from?'

What not to say to someone trying to get pregnant!

'I'm sure you'll get pregnant soon'; 'Trust God more'; 'Have more faith'; 'If it's meant to be it will happen'; 'You could always adopt'; 'At least you still have your husband'; 'His will is best'.

Some of these at least may be true, but they can sound unkind and insensitive.

Also, try to think carefully about rephrasing questions such as, 'Do you have a family?'

For further reading

Lesley Regan, *Miscarriage: What Every Woman Needs to Know*, new edn (Orion, 2001).

Christopher Ash, *Married for God: Making Your Marriage the Best It Can Be* (Inter-Varsity Press, 2007).

HOW CAN THE PROFESSIONALS HELP?

We had to think carefully about whether or not to include this section. We didn't want the aim of this book to be 'How to get a baby', and it looks at first glance as though that is exactly what this section is. However, we are aware that these days if you discuss infertility with anyone at all, the subjects of lifestyle, adoption and, of course, assisted conception will immediately arise. We didn't want Christian people to be left feeling naive when they encounter these conversations. We are also aware that many people facing infertility are in the position of already knowing that the professionals cannot help. You may also already have made the decision not to follow through with treatment or adoption. We do not expect that this section will be relevant to everybody, so please dip into the areas that interest you and disregard the rest! It's also worth pointing out that we are looking at these issues from a UK perspective.

Our main concern is that you are well informed about the options offered by doctors in primary care and by fertility specialists in assisted conception units. We want to prepare you for the decisions facing you if you go forward with treatment or adoption, decisions that will involve careful thought rather than knee-jerk reactions.

What the doctor ordered?

Couples wanting children often find that when others become aware that they are struggling to conceive, they immediately want to know what the doctor's diagnosis is. It is a strange situation to find yourself in, discussing your most intimate details with a relative stranger, particularly when everyone becomes an expert with their various stories of friends who have received successful treatment for assisted conception.

Fiona
Very few people who have got as far as speaking to me about the fact that I am childless have asked me what I think or feel about it. They've focused on the situation, and immediately have gone on to ask me what the medics said (assuming that I've sought medical help) or whether we were going to adopt.

The fact remains that more and more people are going to fertility clinics to help them conceive. In 2007, 13,672 babies were born as a result of IVF treatment, the increasingly common practice of mixing eggs with sperm in a laboratory and implanting the resulting embryos back into the uterus. In Denmark, over 4–5% of the population have been born by IVF.[1] It is a solution that receives a high level of press attention, and most people assume that it will be our first port of call. The fact that only 15–30% of IVF cycles end with a live birth is less widely published. This technology has developed very quickly because there is a massive demand for it, and people are willing to pay huge amounts of money to clinics with good success rates.

In all the hype following the success of IVF and other treatments for assisted conception in the press and among our friends, it is very important to seriously consider the questions that are raised for Christians. We also want to widen the focus and examine other treatments, adoption and ways in which our health and lifestyle may affect fertility.

Underlying this section, however, is a wider concern that some have articulated: 'Should I in faith simply accept infertility as God's will, or do I investigate and have treatment?' Our assumption is that most couples would want to pursue some form of investigation, and we would support that. Infertility is a medical diagnosis, and diagnostic interventions may help to pinpoint the cause. This process will often lead to recommendations for certain treatments, some of which are controversial. In other words, Christians the world over disagree on some of these treatment options. It is not our intention to guide you either for or against specific treatments, or to devote much print to a detailed examination of the options (books such as John Wyatt's *Matters of Life and Death* serve this purpose). Rather, our aim is to highlight questions that will help you carefully to consider all the options. Acceptance of God's will does not rule out investigation and treatment, just as God's sovereignty over the timing of life and death does not lead to ignoring medical help when faced with illness. In his goodness, God has given us doctors and medicine which may be his instruments for healing.

If investigations and treatment do not result in fertility, there may, over time, come a day when a Christian couple accept that their infertility is God's will for them long term. They may then seek guidance as to how else God would have them serve the church, whether through adoption or other ways that do not involve bringing up children. But the timing of acceptance will vary for different people, and it is not an easy process.

When David wrote Psalm 139, it was to praise God for his intimate presence and never-failing control over our lives. The Lord is right there with us, even while we discover the functional failings that he has allowed us to experience. He is there as we work out our way forward in our desire for children.

> I praise you because I am fearfully and wonderfully made;
>> your works are wonderful,
>> I know that full well . . .
> All the days ordained for me
>> were written in your book
>> before one of them came to be.
> (Psalm 139:14, 16b)

11 Lifestyle

Elspeth

When we decided to start a family, my motivation to carry on working as a teacher dropped considerably. I moved schools and went part-time, working three days a week, but the workload that they gave me was huge. As time went on and we weren't conceiving, I considered that perhaps the reason was that I was too stressed and run ragged by the pressures of teaching, travelling, and lack of rest. I rarely ate anything before 4pm because every moment was filled, and I constantly caught colds, developed infections and experienced regular bouts of cystitis. I would fall asleep on the sofa when I came home from work and yet be buzzing in the middle of the night, unable to sleep. I didn't want to consider that this pace of life was preventing us from having a baby, but looking back I can't help wondering if it had a big effect on me. I guess I'll never know.

Assessing your lifestyle

When you hear stories of people who seem to get pregnant in the most unhealthy and stressful of situations, it can be frustrating to consider that your own fertility may be affected by your current lifestyle. There is no conclusive evidence to prove that lifestyle issues such as sleep, exercise and diet are direct reasons for infertility. But research carried out by the National Health Service and by many natural therapy practitioners has found some links. It must be stressed that this is inconclusive. Therefore, in considering lifestyle, we need to realize that we are helping ourselves to cope with our situation in more ways than one. Our mental and emotional faculties may draw on all the physical strength we have as we face the stresses of infertility.

In a busy world where work can swallow us up, as Elspeth is finding, it is easy to lose sight of basic ways of keeping yourself healthy. The following list of questions is just meant as a quick checklist to highlight any areas that are draining you in ways that you hadn't noticed before.

- Are you sleeping well? What steps can you take to get the sleep you need?
- Do you get enough exercise?
- Are you eating a balanced diet with plenty of essential vitamins?
- Does your alcohol intake need reducing?
- Are there any excessive emotional tensions in your life and are they avoidable?

It may be that you are up against factors that make it impossible to improve your health and stress levels, so you mustn't feel that you are already failing if your lifestyle is far from perfect! If you need guidance on making your lifestyle a bit healthier, ask a doctor or a nutritionist to see if they can spot any obvious problems. They can then help you to correct them so that you are as healthy as possible as you attempt to conceive.

Catherine
It's amazing the lengths we went to in our campaign to have a baby.
I joined a Rosemary Conley diet club and lost almost 20 kg in weight
on a low-fat diet, and Luke joined me and lost a considerable amount
of weight too. Having healthier bodies and for Luke, wearing loose
boxer shorts and having cold showers all gave us hope that we might
conceive. We didn't immediately, but even so, I think that losing the
excess weight was good for us.

As a couple you may have to be very patient with each other while you are investigating possibilities, particularly if they are not cheap. It may be that wives become far more proactive in taking up suggestions offered by friends about clinics, diets, exercise routines and alternative therapies. They may go ahead and make appointments with doctors and therapists about issues concerning what is going on in their body and in their mind. A wife may get frustrated when her husband doesn't seem to be doing anything apart from making sarcastic comments about her ideas. He may just want to get her to wait or to discuss things at the right time, but she may interpret this as cynicism or, worse still, an unwillingness to work at making it possible for them to have children. Remember that husband and wife will inevitably move at different speeds. Give each other the chance to get used to new ideas and try to discuss them before doing anything rash.

Consideration for the little guys

This is the part where we go into details that may endanger the spontaneity of lovemaking! We have decided to include this information simply because you may not have come across it elsewhere. If you have already read about keeping sperm alive then skip the following paragraph! It comes as advice from a medical friend.

It may be useful to reflect on factors that can affect sperm production and motility. The male body is designed so that sperm are produced and stored at a lower temperature than the man's core body temperature. The temperature of the scrotum can be raised too high, endangering sperm, if the man takes baths that are too hot, wears tight-fitting underwear or sits in the same position for long periods of time. The motility and function of sperm can also be affected by lubricant gels and creams, as well as soaps used for douching. A man carries the healthiest amount of sperm if he abstains from ejaculation for three or four days. Abstaining for fewer than twenty-four hours will produce a below-optimum amount. Sperm will have the best chance of making it through the cervical mucus if there is deep penetration at the start of the ejaculation.

Monitoring ovulation

Most women are able to identify when they are likely to start a period, and some may even have physical symptoms accompanying ovulation. Their moods may swing up about ten days after a period has come and swing down a few days before its next appearance. Periods may arrive with such regularity that the critical days on which pregnancy might occur can be pinpointed accurately and the necessary arrangements made! However, for those with irregular or very long cycles, monitoring ovulation can be a long process. There are a variety of hormones that can be tested for to find out what stage of the cycle you have got to and to establish that you have the right levels of hormones at each point in your cycle. You can read about hormones and the menstrual cycle in more detail on websites concerned with women's health and fertility. They will help you to understand the details of the menstrual cycle and the physical changes that accompany each stage. These hormones are present in blood, saliva and urine samples. Some can be detected only by blood tests, but others, such as the LH (luteinizing hormone) surge before ovulation, can be tested by urine test-sticks.

Natural fertility treatments

Alongside the growth in reproductive technology has come a recent upsurge in the use of natural fertility treatments that focus on a woman's natural cycle. These involve teaching women to monitor their hormones and other biomarkers during their own ovulatory cycles. Irregularities may indicate the need for non-invasive treatment or medication. The aim of natural fertility is to make the physiological conditions that are necessary for pregnancy as near perfect as possible. Great wisdom and patience are needed as we find out about alternative methods of fertility treatment that may help us. We are extremely vulnerable emotionally and financially, and the appeal of these treatments and new ideas may sweep us along a particular path too hastily. We need to be most concerned for our spiritual health and put our trust in God's control, so that we don't just rely on the power of our practitioner.

Search me, O God, and know my heart;
    test me and know my anxious thoughts.
See if there is any offensive way in me,
    and lead me in the way everlasting.
(Psalm 139:23–24)

An initial visit to the doctor

If you have no knowledge of factors that may inhibit your fertility, and the woman is under the age of thirty-five, in the UK it is recommended that you wait about a year before going to your doctor. When the woman is thirty-five or over, a doctor will see you after six months.

Some people would like to know what will happen if they go to a doctor saying that they are unable to conceive naturally. He or she will assume that you have been having regular unprotected sex during that time and will ask questions about both of your histories and present state of health. Problems may have arisen from illnesses in the past, such as cancer and its associated treatments, chronic infections, anaemia, metabolic or hormonal problems which may have left you with fertility issues. You may be on a course of drugs that may also impair your fertility, such as steroids, anti-malarials or those used to treat urinary infections or depression. Your doctor may also want to ensure that you have an accurate understanding of the days in the month when you are most likely to conceive and give you some of the health advice mentioned already.

Kath

I always knew that having children would be difficult for me because I was diagnosed with polycystic ovary syndrome (PCOS) when I was sixteen. I knew that someday, in order to conceive, medical intervention would be needed to encourage me to ovulate. Without help I would have ovulated and had a period once a year. So far my treatment has included taking the medication Clomid, which did not have much effect. This was followed by a laparoscopy, hysteroscopy and multi-puncture diathermy operation (an operation giving slight burns to the ovaries that is meant to stimulate them to ovulate) which made me ovulate once, but I have not ovulated since.

I am now back on Clomid to see if the operation and Clomid together can stimulate ovulation. If not, then it will be Clomid and Metformin together, then Clomid and injections together. If this fails then the next step would be IVF.

I have found the hospital treatment very clinical and have sometimes felt like a specimen. The treatment is very intrusive and emotionally draining. There are prods and pokes, cameras, scans, blood tests, questions and more questions. There are lectures on anatomy, diet, weight, regularity of sex, menstrual cycle and on it goes. There are expectations, discouragements and confusion. However, we do have a loving and caring Christian infertility consultant. We are so grateful to God for her and that she always directs us to pray. We are then reminded that no matter what medical treatment says, we have a God who can ordain whatever he wills.

After an initial visit to the doctor, you will probably be referred to your nearest fertility unit for investigative tests. These will include some blood tests to establish that ovulation is occurring and a sperm sample test to ensure that sperm are motile and sufficient in number. The results of these tests may bring issues to light. It may be that they are able to identify specific problems that lie with one or both of you. On the other hand, they may simply throw up more questions than answers. The results may be devastating and conclusive in their verdict in cases where sperm or eggs are simply not being produced. However, more often, the results present couples with further decisions to make.

Mary

I was diagnosed with an early menopause about eighteen months ago. I went to my doctor because my periods were absent after coming off the pill. My husband and I had been married for a few years and I had stopped taking the pill with the aim of starting a family. The doctor did some initial blood tests and I was referred to a fertility consultant. After further tests, they concluded that essentially my ovaries were no longer producing eggs, and that I had pre-ovulation failure or an early menopause. I think initially I was expecting that this meant there was still a chance that I could become pregnant naturally, but over time I realized that this was not likely. My care changed to the early menopause clinic. I was offered counselling, as well as access to various support groups, and I have been seeing the counsellor. This service has been excellent.

IUI (intra-uterine insemination)

When we went for tests, both of us (Eleanor and Sue) were told that we had unexplained infertility. As couples we had all the relevant investigative tests but there was nothing wrong with our results. Everything worked fine. There were no obvious reasons as to why we weren't getting pregnant. We were advised to keep trying naturally or to go ahead with IUI as a stepping stone to IVF.

Tom

We were offered IVF but we felt very uncomfortable at the thought of creating a number of embryos and having to discard some. We did opt for IUI and had three cycles of treatment at a large teaching hospital in London. Rachel took hormones to boost ovulation and I'd provided sperm to be treated by the clinic who would rouse the troops. I would take my pot over to the clinic and dump it into what looked like a large free-standing ashtray outside the lab. On one occasion I was delayed so I phoned to explain. 'I have my sperm sample ready but I'm running late, so should I do another?' A male voice answered, 'Can I stop you there, mate, you've come through to the press room of the Mirror *newspaper!'*

IUI works in a similar way to the traditional artificial insemination, with some medical advances thrown in. It tracks the woman's cycle and boosts egg production, using hormones taken by tablet or injection. She is scanned two or three times in the second week of her cycle to monitor the growth of the follicles on her ovaries, as well as assessing the thickness and quality of the womb lining. When the LH hormone is produced, signalling the onset of ovulation, the couple come into the unit. The man produces a sperm sample which is treated to produce the best possible concentration of sperm, and this is injected up into the woman's cervix. Two weeks later you take a pregnancy test and phone the unit to let them know the result for their records. Soon after that the bill arrives.

Christine
The tests and the laparoscopy were inconclusive, so the verdict was 'unexplained infertility'. I had three cycles of IUI treatment, all accompanied by a course of Clomid. I felt that my treatment by the staff was always rather off-hand, and I kept being given wrong instructions so that the tablets or injections were not taken or given at the right times.

Up until about five years ago IUI had a success rate of 12%, while the IVF rate was closer to 20%. IUI is popular with couples because it is cheaper, irons out any potentially basic problems and does not involve surgery. Today, most doctors may see little point in spending any funding on IUI because it is regarded as too low-tech. As a result, they may push couples more insistently towards IVF. It is interesting to note that where funding is available for infertile couples, they are funded to do IVF, not IUI. Results of pregnancies are important for a fertility unit. If they can publish a higher rate of success, then they will gain a higher place in the league tables, attracting more funding and more clients.

We both liked the idea of IUI because, as well as costing less, it meant that we could hold off thinking about the bigger issues linked to IVF. It was also a way of ensuring that all of the factors necessary for conception were absolutely in place. However, in our cases it also brought disappointment and frustration.

12 Treatment

Forty years ago, if you couldn't conceive, then the only real medical option open to you was artificial insemination or donor insemination. Things have changed quite a bit since then and are still changing. Ever since the birth of the first 'test-tube' baby, Louise Brown, on 25 July 1978, the use of *in vitro* fertilization or IVF technology has given childless couples a reason to hope for the child that they could not otherwise have. The real possibility that grew out of this development was that problems inside the body could be overcome by realizing a conception outside it. Although IVF was first used in the case of a woman who had blocked Fallopian tubes, this technology, developed by embryologist Dr Patrick Steptoe and gynaecologist Dr Robert Edwards, was to go on to make many more options possible for a range of difficulties. IVF literally means 'fertilization in a dish' and puts the man's sperm together with eggs harvested from the woman's ovaries to create a single cell which then begins to divide, known at this early stage as the 'embryo'. A few of the strongest-looking embryos are chosen to be inserted into the womb, where they will hopefully implant and develop normally in the same way as a natural conception. The remaining embryos can then be frozen cryogenically, to be used by the couple at a later date, donated to research, donated to another couple or discarded. If the sperm are not strong enough to fuse with the egg, a single sperm can be injected into the egg in a process known as 'intracytoplasmic sperm injection' (ICSI).

The UK National Infertility Awareness Campaign published a report back in 1998 which led to the recommendation by NICE (National Institute of Clinical Excellence) that all health-care trusts should fund at least one cycle of IVF for infertile couples under the age of forty. As a result, British primary care trusts are now meant to offer between one and three funded cycles of fertility treatment but these tend to be accompanied by long waiting lists and strict access criteria. Although the infertility network website provides support and counselling for infertile couples, its main concern is to get couples the funding they need to proceed with IVF.

Thinking through IVF for yourself

Doctors are incredibly busy and pressured, and they are guided in their practice by the questions, 'Is this course of treatment possible?' and 'Is it safe for you?' They are not necessarily going to be concerned with the question, 'Is this okay for you as a Christian?' If the treatment that could help you is legal and suits your situation, then they will recommend that you follow it up. They will usually advise that you proceed sooner rather than later, since the age of the woman has an influence on the success of the treatment.

If you long for a baby, these pressures may cause you to consent to a course of action without thinking much about the implications. You may understandably be very excited by a treatment that could help to end your pain, but the momentum created by those explanations and statistics in a doctor's surgery may be difficult to stop in its tracks once you have begun down that line. It is so much better to work out your boundaries and values before you get to the consulting room.

For Christians, it is not an understatement to say that IVF is an extremely controversial issue. Although we want to help couples as they face childlessness and try to cope with the pressures that this brings, we are not medics or ethicists, and feel distinctly lacking in the ability to guide you in detail through these questions. John Wyatt in *Matters of Life and Death* deals with these issues with the necessary knowledge, wisdom and experience. In chapter 3, 'Reproductive technology and the start of life', he identifies the key areas to consider, holding the Christian faith and the relevant medical processes in an intelligent tension. In chapter 7, 'When is a person? Christian perspectives on the beginning of life', he explores the biblical material on the distinctions between the early stages of conception and the later foetus.

Wyatt also references several other texts on the subject and is a good springboard to further research. An Internet search on 'the Christian ethics of IVF' and similar keyword searches will also return articles and websites for consideration.

As a starting point to your research, we would like to introduce you to two of the questions at the heart of the debate, questions we feel are essential for any couple considering the possibility of assisted conception. It is not our purpose explicitly to condemn or condone any one course of action, because we recognize that people differ. However, we want to be unambiguous about the central issues and to stress their implications. In simply asking these questions, we may well come across as being for or against in these matters. If this is the case, we hope that you will still be able to research and prayerfully wrestle with the issues for yourself and to draw conclusions that you are content to live with.

> **Peter and Vivienne**
> *It is one thing to debate the ethics of infertility treatment when it isn't your own problem, but when you are confronted with potential childlessness, the need for a definite way forward, and the hope it gives, the issue is much more pressing. We opted to pursue IVF: we appreciate that other Christian couples can and do choose not to.*

Question 1: What is the status of the early embryo?

'For you created my inmost being; you knit me together in my mother's womb' (Psalm 139:13). Have you ever wondered when life begins exactly? Some believe that life begins at the point of conception, when the sperm first fuses with the egg. Others argue that it is only after the embryo is implanted into the wall of the uterus, when an umbilical cord is formed and the blood of the mother begins to sustain it, that a functional new life can begin.

The answer to this question will determine our attitude to the practice of embryo selection that is at the heart of IVF treatment. If a pre-implanted embryo is indeed a new life, then Christians will not want to 'discard' it because, in doing so, we take the place of God in deciding to end that life. Even if we freeze embryos for use at a future date, we cannot absolutely guarantee that all of them will eventually be implanted.

Beth
All too often, I have spoken to people who just haven't thought through the issue. It strikes me that for the generation I was brought up in, this question was a very important one, but IVF is so celebrated today, that I think many people would listen to the media, and not even think to engage with the issue. Personally I feel quite strongly about life beginning at conception, and so for us, IVF was never an option.

We need to take this issue seriously and do our research on the status of the early embryo before we embark on treatment. Thankfully we are not on our own in this matter, and we recommend looking not only at John Wyatt's book but also at the Christian Medical Fellowship website, where you will find articles on reproductive technologies by experts such as Peter Saunders.[2] These ethicists are also medics who deem it of the utmost importance to retain a high level of respect and compassion for those who find themselves in the position of having to make such decisions.

Question 2: If I accept donor eggs or sperm, am I introducing a third person into my marriage? How will a resulting child view his or her identity?

For those who cannot produce their own eggs or sperm, there is another difficult decision to face: whether or not to accept eggs or sperm from a donor. Christians will want to think through this carefully because of the importance of the marriage covenant. Many consider that the unique blend of the two persons of a married couple into the one genetic child is violated by the introduction of the physical presence of a third person. Others view the resulting child as a product of the parents' love, whatever his or her genetic make-up. The medics we encounter are not paid to take us through the ethical considerations from a Christian point of view. We must do this work for ourselves.

> **Mary**
> *In terms of fertility options, egg donation and adoption were quite easily introduced by the professionals, without really emphasizing the complexities involved in these choices. I personally had a strong feeling that egg donation was not an option for us, and that a child would not be a union of us as a couple.*

The issue of donors is also controversial because of the questions that are raised for the resulting child. This child may question, when told of the circumstances of his or her conception, what it means to be the product of one parent and not the other, and may also ask questions about the absent genetic 'parent', particularly when doctors ask about conditions running in the family. Since the Human Fertilisation and Embryology Bill in 2008, it has become necessary for the details of donors giving sperm, eggs or embryos to be made available to the couple and subsequently to the child. This means that donors are increasingly difficult to find, because they face the possibility of a future knock on the door from someone who has been conceived using their sperm or egg. There is also no financial recompense, which makes the prospect of undergoing the potentially dangerous enterprise of providing eggs almost unthinkable for a woman, no matter how altruistic she is feeling. The usual course of action is for fertility clinics to offer free or reduced-price cycles of treatment in return for surplus eggs, sperm and embryos. This can potentially enable those without sufficient funds to undergo treatment.

The issues surrounding the question of whether and how to tell the child of his or her parentage are also profoundly different from those for an adopted or stepchild. With regard to adoption or stepchildren, the chief concerns are about the parenting arrangements and the rights of an existing child. The best interests of the child and his or her future perception of the past and identity are given great consideration. In the case of a child conceived using donor eggs or sperm, these issues are not even considered. The chief concerns are about the best interests and rights of the parents.

Annie and Jack

We finally found out what the problem was and were then referred to the fertility clinic at the hospital. The appointment came through very fast and we found ourselves sitting in front of a consultant, who just stated that the option available to us in our circumstances was to have a donor. At no point in the conversation with the consultant did he ask us how we felt emotionally about using a donor; it was just assumed that we would do anything to have a baby. He wanted to get started straightaway, but we stopped him and said we needed to go away and think about what he was suggesting as an option for us. When we got home, we felt as though we were being pushed down a route without any prayer or thoughts regarding the donor. We discussed 'the donor' a lot and, in the end, we both felt that it would be clouded in secrecy for the child and, if the truth ever came out, the child would have a huge emotional struggle to work through. We went back to prayer, asking God whether this would be right or not; this was something we wanted, but that didn't necessarily mean that children were part of God's plan for our lives. After much prayer and talking to each other, we decided to take ourselves off the fertility clinic's list: we felt it was very materialistic and not for us. Instead, we turned our focus back to God and asked for his help and guidance. I prayed to him that if he didn't mean us to have children, he would give me a peace of mind over this. The peace of mind did come. At times, it has been severely tested, but through the prayers of our friends it has returned.

Of course, it is so easy to slip into a discussion of this topic without considering what it is actually like to be in the position of making such a decision. Annie and Jack's experience shows the agony of saying 'no', not just once, but time and time again. John Wyatt ends his chapter on reproductive technologies with a reminder that, if couples decide not to go ahead with treatments because of their convictions, they are making a big sacrifice and need support from other Christians around them.

> By refraining from reproductive technology, a childless couple may bear witness to God's creation order while having to pay the price of exclusion from part of the blessings of that order. As a Christian community, we should learn to recognize and honour the painful sacrifice which such couples make.[1]

Craig
Our families are anxious that we should try everything possible to have a child. They can't understand why we want to think through everything so much, particularly with regard to IVF. They said that they didn't want to pressurize us, but we absolutely knew what they thought. My wife's mum was more worried about her daughter's health and what all the treatments might do to her. We found that we had become experts on it all, and many people don't know what they're talking about. You want to say, 'Look, I have actually thought about this. I'm not just trying to be difficult. If we thought it was fine then obviously we would be doing this. We're just not convinced yet.' Many of our friends and family are thoughtful in so many ways as Christians, but this is such a new invention that they just haven't engaged with it yet.

Like any other difficult ethical issue, it would be wonderful just to be told what we should do in a given situation. We are well aware that this section may leave you with far more questions than answers. We hope that setting out the issues in this way will help to challenge you to consider your options now, rather than have to face unforeseen complications and regrets later on in life.

13 Adoption?

Beth

I felt full of hope when I filled in the application form. My heart was set on adoption. I had realized that the opportunity of adopting a young child was unlikely and that there were fewer white children available for adoption, so we would be in a minority, but still I was undeterred.

The word 'adopt' comes from the Latin *adoptare* which means 'to choose'. To adopt is to take by choice a child who has not been born to you into relationship in your family and to treat him or her as your own. There is much to say on the subject of adoption and we are aware that a single chapter will not do it justice. We hope that you will find it useful as an introduction to the issues that it can involve, even though it does not comprehensively cover all of the stages and potential complications of the process. It's worth a reminder here that, as far as the adoption processes go, we are coming from a UK perspective. But we hope the overarching issues that adoption raises for Christians will be helpful to all.

Eleanor

After our three cycles of IUI had failed, we gave ourselves a set period of time during which we decided to put off thinking about having children. We were worn out with the emotional roller coaster of the previous four years. We set a date when we thought we would be ready to start thinking about adoption. For us, adoption was the obvious next step. Nick and his brother and sister were all adopted, as were two of my cousins. We had close friends who were adopted, and friends at church had just adopted their daughter. These experiences of adoption were very varied, with some great successes and others bringing many difficulties. Nevertheless, despite people talking us through some of the negative sides of adoption, we decided to apply to our local authority to be assessed as potential adopters.

What is the adoption process like?

The process of adoption is not quick, but in the UK there are far fewer restrictions on *who* can adopt than there were fifteen years ago. Experiences of the adoption process vary enormously and often depend on the quality of the personal attention offered by particular social workers and adoption agencies. You can choose to adopt through government-run agencies, adoption charities or international agencies.

Eleanor

We found the whole process of adoption tremendously exciting and very difficult at the same time. At the start, we were overwhelmed by the difference in the attitude of the professionals who we were dealing with in our local authority. Instead of the consumer-based approach of the fertility clinic, we were being welcomed and valued as people who were doing something extremely positive for an existing child needing a permanent home.

Andrew and Beth

We decided to pursue adoption and felt very positive about our decision. An introductory evening with our local council didn't fill us with confidence. It was led by a social worker who sadly lacked any social skills. It was one of the most painful evenings that I have ever attended. Despite this, we worked through the paperwork and felt very positive. We received a letter (printed upside down on their headed paper) saying that we had to apply for a child of four or five years old or we would not be considered. I felt mortified. At no point during the introductory evening were we told this. Our experience of speaking to 'private' adoption agencies has been completely different. They listened to us and got to know us. It was a personal process which gave us great confidence.

Trevor and Stacey

We went to a meeting run by an international adoption agency. They talked about orphanages abroad where one nurse was in charge of far too many babies. We saw the potential for Western couples to provide these children with a lifetime of love instead of the neglect that they currently face. This agency said that they would complete the home study with us themselves, so that we did not have to go through our local council. They also knew exactly what the legal requirements would be, and could help us through all those stages that we felt were beyond us. We think that we will probably look more into adoption closer to home, but it was really useful to get an international perspective.

Obviously it is best to find an adoption agency who you feel are listening to you and providing you with the answers and support that you need. You will need to have a good working relationship with them through all of the interviews and decision-making that lie ahead.

Eleanor

Our home study (the procedure to assess the suitability of those wanting to adopt) was very quick, taking about six months to complete. It comprised of thirty-five to forty hours or so of interviews with our assigned social worker. We got on very well with her and enjoyed the sessions, which were regular meetings each lasting about two hours. The aim of these sessions was to gather sufficient information about us to ensure that we were suitable as adopters and to delve into every aspect of our own experiences of being parented, our past relationships and our current lifestyle, family structure, friendships, beliefs and value systems. At times it felt like our social worker was writing our biographies! The resulting document was a sixty-page dossier known as a Form F, which contained all the information needed to prove that we were able and ready to adopt and which gave a good impression of the home that we could provide for a child.

Andrew and Beth

Unfortunately for us the timescale was wrong. They needed us to commit to more than two years for the adoption process, and at the time we thought we would have to move during this period and couldn't guarantee being in their catchment area. So sadly we were turned down. Although this was upsetting, the manner in which we were treated was exceptional and softened the bad news.

Who are the children available for adoption today?

Before the wide availability of the Pill and easy access to abortion, many babies were available for adoption because their mothers got pregnant at a young age and generally had to give them up for social or religious reasons. Today, the emphasis in local authorities is strongly on birth mothers keeping their babies and working at the problems of a young mother coping with a child. This means that the children available for adoption today are generally those who cannot stay with their birth mothers, either because they and the family do not wish to take care of them, such as in the case of severe disability, or because of actual or threatened forms of abuse or neglect.

Although the situations of many children available for adoption make them difficult to place, it is important to stress that adopters are free to choose whom they adopt. One of the first forms that we filled in asked us to indicate what sort of physical, emotional and background factors we would or would not be able to cope with when considering a child. We weren't held to it and were free to change our minds further down the line, but it gave our social worker a good idea of what sort of child we envisaged adopting. Agency websites and news bulletins display profiles of children who are available for adoption, but they are often those who are termed as 'hard to place'. It is possible to adopt under-fives and 'uncomplicated' children, but you are less likely to see their profiles because their cases move much more quickly, as you will find if you are matched with them.

Peter and Heather

We were very pleased to be told that it was more important to recognize the benefit the children would be to us rather than the benefit we would be to the children. In other words, our need of them was as great as their need of us. This gave us a sense of gratitude and respect for them, which counteracts any sense of our 'doing good' to them and giving them an exaggerated sense of obligation to us.

How does a child move from foster care to an adoptive placement?

Foster care may at first be regarded as a temporary placement while the initial problems with the child's birth family are addressed. The emphasis is on lots of contact visits by the mother, and the route to reconciliation is always pursued as the highest good. However, when it has been decided by social workers that there is no hope of the child being looked after satisfactorily by his or her mother, the court issues a freeing order which allows a placement for adoption to be sought. It is at this point that social workers seek a match with approved adopters. After the agreement of the matching panel, contact with the foster family and the child begins and a series of visits works towards the child going home with the adopters.

Reflections of a foster parent

Many of the babies we looked after went on to be adopted. After the first visit we would encourage the adopters to increase their interaction by changing, feeding, playing and settling for the night. Over the next few days (or sometimes weeks) they would take the child out for the day. At first these were with us present, then later unaccompanied. Next came visits to the new home. We would accompany for the first visit, to show the child that we were happy to be in the new home, and later the child would visit without us. Then comes moving-on day. These occasions were a mixture of feelings for us. Sad to be losing 'our' child, but happy that he or she had found a 'forever' family.

Once the child has gone home with the adoptive parents, the arrangement is termed as 'placed for adoption', since the child is still a 'looked-after child' under the responsibility of social services. Visits from a variety of social workers continue until the adoption panel hearing, after which the child legally becomes the son or daughter of the adopting couple. This is the point at which the birth certificate is issued with the names of the adoptive couple on it.

How can Christians be confident in the adoption process?

Eleanor

Throughout our home study we made it very clear that we were committed Christians. Nick's job as a youth worker and the time that we spent on church activities meant that we were questioned about our beliefs and lifestyle in some detail. The social workers were keen to find out how our faith would impact a child living in our family. We were asked at every stage about how we would feel if our adopted child decided not to believe as we did, or if he or she lived a lifestyle that was at odds with our faith.

Many Christians are concerned that social workers will be suspicious of their faith and church activities. There may well be stories that you have heard that involve the prejudices of a given social worker making it difficult for a couple to proceed. They could certainly pick on a detail that we had thought of as insignificant and make it a key reason as to why we would be unsuitable.

But we discovered that committed Christians can actually talk about their faith in such a way that it puts them at a real advantage as adopters. We can also use potentially difficult moments in the home study, such as those times when we are questioned about our thoughts on alternative lifestyles. We can demonstrate that, alongside our faith in the words of the Bible, we are realistic enough to be in touch with the way in which the world works and have experience of working peacefully and graciously with different world-views in our lives, even when we disagree with them.

Love is a decision

Christians can also be confident in going forward for adoption because we are taught to take love seriously. The promise to love is widely misunderstood in society today. God's promise to love Israel and then to love those who trust in Christ is a promise that he commits to, even when we don't love him back. This example of covenant love is one that we are familiar with in marriage and it is true for adoption too. We may be flooded by love and compassion when we first look at a photo of a child and read about him or her, or meet for the first time. At that point we may feel that this child deserves our love because of all that he or she has been through and because the child has been given a poor start in life. Our love will grow and develop as with any relationship, but those same feelings of compassion may well not be present when we hit tough times. The child does not receive our love because he or she deserves it, but because we have decided from the beginning to love him or her. When we adopt a child, we do not have to follow set words, but we are promising to continue to love, even when things get really horrible. We are promising by a deliberate action to give this child all the status and privileges of being part of our family, no matter what. We will care, provide and make sacrifices for this child, and he or she will inherit all that we have alongside any other children we may have.

God talks in Hosea about the sacrifice of loving Israel as an adoptive son:

> It was I who taught Ephraim to walk,
>   taking them by the arms;
> but they did not realise
>   it was I who healed them.

I led them with cords of human kindness,
  with ties of love;
I lifted the yoke from their neck
  and bent down to feed them.
(Hosea 11:3–4)

In the Christian world, there are many stories of adoptions that have brought hurt and troubled times to the family. These are normal families with ordinary lives and faithful, loving parents, who have had to bear more than their non-adoptive contemporaries because they have had to battle with factors that are quite definitely out of their control. These factors include drug-taking during pregnancy, abusive treatment in the early years, the deep-rooted effect of being moved between birth parents and foster placements, neglect that has caused communication issues and developmental delay. Adoptive parents spend a lot of time wondering how much is nature and how much is nurture. The temptation is to blame any ambiguities on the adoption, but the reality is that an adopted child is not a blank canvas, and we have signed up from the beginning, not just for a child to relieve our childlessness, but for a human being who requires our unconditional love.

Heather

It is vital for the adoptive parents really to have come to terms with their childlessness. At our first interview with our adoption agency, I was asked how I felt about being barren! I was a bit shocked at the directness of the question, but it helped me enormously to face that fact. This has subsequently been very helpful when things became difficult. The question of nature versus nurture was something I didn't really face at the time of adopting Edward. We were told he had a very different background from Maria, but I did not think that

would matter, as I felt that our love for him would outweigh
everything! How wrong I was, and looking back I think we should
have done more to understand his background.

We are adopted people

The Bible tells us that by nature we do not belong to God's family. When Paul talks to the Galatians, he describes the Christian as someone whose status has been radically changed. The Christian is taken into God's family at great cost, because of the death of Jesus. 'So you are no longer a slave, but a son; and since you are a son, God has made you also an heir' (Galatians 4:7).

The whole story of the Bible is God's plan of salvation that brings us from being his enemies to being his children. He makes us his children to the extent that we are brothers and sisters of Christ and share an inheritance together with him of the riches and treasures of heaven. We know peace with God and are promised eternity with him, just as if we were Jesus himself.

So we know the value of being adopted. It is of massive benefit to us personally. In being able to extend that benefit to another human being, we are reflecting the passions of God's own heart. 'In love he predestined us to be adopted as his sons through Jesus Christ, in accordance with his pleasure and will' (Ephesians 1:4b–5). We are mirroring God's image and doing something that is a truly godly action. We learn more of who God is and what he is like when we adopt a child who is not naturally ours and treat that child as we would treat our biological children.

At our adoption preparation classes we met a Christian adoptive family who had never had fertility problems, but who had simply decided that since God had adopted them, they would do the same for others. They didn't make a great song and dance about it, but social services were using them as a demonstration family who came in and told us about their experiences. They had even borne the stigma of misunderstanding when they adopted a three-year-old child when they had been married for only two years.

Our status does not depend on passing on our genes

Catherine

I remember doing some gardening one day with my mother and having a chat about the possibility of adopting a child. We had been looking into adoption and fertility treatment by this time. Luke was not keen to embark on fertility treatment, so we were investigating our options through adoption agencies. My mother made a comment about having your own child as being the most desirable thing, if we could. It felt like a stab through the heart, like what I was trying to 'offer her' was not good enough. I know she meant well, but it hurt to hear it.

I wonder how often people have commented on how much you look like your mother or father. As I (Eleanor) have grown older, I have been compared more and more to my mother, particularly by my aunt. I often hear my mother's voice as I talk, particularly when I am teaching. It is fun to identify facial features and mannerisms that run in families, but it would be so sad if these were the only things that generated love between family members.

Many people object to adoption because they don't want to have a child with a different genetic make-up from their own. While I can understand the desire for a package of DNA that is familiar to us, I would also like gently to challenge this notion. What do we most want to pass on to others in our lives as Christians? Surely it is not the shape of our nose. Paul, an unmarried, childless man, talked about his desire to see spiritual understanding and God-honouring lives in those he taught, those who were as dear to him as sons and daughters. Christian parents are taught to bring their young ones up in the fear and instruction of the Lord (Deuteronomy 31:12–13), and we trust that he will show no less mercy to those that we have not given birth to than he does to those we have.

We will be non-judgmental regarding the failings of birth parents

It is important to social workers involved in adoption that adopters are able to talk about the birth parents of their adopted child without prejudice. This is because it is tempting to want to paint a very negative picture so that the child realizes how important it was to be moved to be part of your family.

When we were looking at the profiles of children available for adoption, we were able to ask for the details of those who particularly caught our attention. As we read through the files of these children, it quickly became clear that their birth parents were guilty of a range of mistakes, some accidental and some quite deliberate, that would have a serious impact on the children for the rest of their lives. Other people, including us, would have to spend a great deal of time and energy undoing the harm that they had inflicted on their children. At times, reading about their actions made us extremely angry and very sad, and led us to question how God could have allowed these people to become parents in the first place. As Christians, however, we understand forgiveness, since we ourselves have been forgiven. We may not have manifested the types of sin that we have read about, but Jesus' own assessment of the severity of any sin, whether thought or acted out, means that we are no 'better' than them. Our comments about them to our adopted child will reflect this understanding, at the same time as explaining the need for the child to have been moved. Great wisdom is needed and your social worker will be pleased to see your concern for this to be done well. The child will need to understand the need for the move, but will also need to have God's forgiveness modelled for him or her in the attitude of the adoptive parents.

Church – a great support network!

We should not be ashamed of belonging to a church and being involved. It provides much of the community and care that many people feel are lacking in our modern society. The church has traditionally been recognized as providing care for the poor and disabled, the slave and the orphan, well before the welfare system and social workers were committed to this work. In that sense we are working on the same team as our social workers, and our attitude will be less defensive if we can see them in this light.

One of the exercises we had to do as part of the home study was to draw a diagram showing the friends and family who would support us in the process of adoption. It is important to social services that we have really great friends who will help us when things get difficult. Our church family is a ready-made dream support network. There we have people who will sacrifice their time, energy and money in their support of us as we pursue adoption.

Adoption should not be rushed into

Tom and Rachel

We did look into adoption, but as health-care professionals we were being steered towards children with complex needs, and we

increasingly felt that we didn't want our home to become an
extension of work. Our marriage was also under enormous strain,
and I felt that realistically we could not take on a challenge like this.

Adoption is not for everyone, and this section is not designed to pressurize Christians into going into it without serious thought as to how it might affect them and their subsequent family. Sometimes, just beginning the process of adoption may confirm that the right path for you as a couple is not to adopt.

Reflecting on chapters 11 – 13

Something to read

How are Christians challenged to live as we make decisions? Read Psalm 40, particularly verse 8, 'I desire to do your will, O my God; your law is within my heart', and the whole of Romans 12, particularly verse 12, 'Be joyful in hope, patient in affliction, faithful in prayer.'

Something to do

Keep a diary or journal as you go through different treatments or the adoption process. Record your highs and lows alongside your reflections on God's Word. Keep commenting on sermons you have heard, things Christian friends have told you, your own Bible reading and study with others, so that they will keep you rooted in God's priorities and in the knowledge of his care for you.

A conversation to have

Whatever course of action you would like to take requires careful thought. Set aside time as a couple to discuss the relevant issues and plan when you are going to do your research and approximately how long you are going to leave between treatments.

For friends and pastors

Ask the couple what you can be praying for at this particular stage of the process. In addition to their prayer requests, pray on your own that the couple will be content and trust God and his provision for them, whatever the outcome of the process. Ask them what might cause them hope or disappointment along the way. Each meeting or appointment will bring further issues to pray about.

For further reading

To think more about the issues surrounding IVF, have a look at John Wyatt's book *Matters of Life and Death* (Inter-Varsity Press, 2009), especially chapter 3, 'Reproductive technology and the start of life', and chapter 7, 'When is a person?'

SECTION 4:

THE LONG UNKNOWN

14 Is acceptance possible?

Kath

I generally feel pessimistic about whether we will ever have children, but I know that I have to remember that God is in control. It is very difficult to remember this continually, and it is the last thing I want to hear from someone else, but I know that this is the only thing that will keep me going and strengthen my faith.

When we (Sue and Steve) were first married, we were friends with a couple who had been trying to conceive for ten years. When they told us this, I remember feeling sorry for them, thinking, Why don't they just accept that this is not going to happen? After all, ten years! It's a long time! Why don't they just accept what seems to be inevitable? And here I am, seventeen years into a childless marriage, realizing that the hope doesn't ever really go away. It may vary in intensity with different women and men, but as one of my friends put it, infertility is a chronic grief: the long unknown.

With the passage of time comes a dawning realization that I am not going to have a child. You don't arrive at this point suddenly one day. It is something you glide in to, something that creeps up on you. Coming to the end of the road of tests and procedures brings with it a weight: a weight of the finality of God's choice for you. Time has run out. The truth sinks in a little further. It is no longer physically possible to bear children, even if I have all the money, time and medical help to try and conceive.

This is another stage in the grief process. I have to come to terms with the thought that this might be God's will for my 'best'. I can no longer hold out hope that next month might be just the month that I miss my period. The response to well-meaning enquiries changes from 'Well, we're trying', to 'No, we haven't been able to have children.' Hearing myself say that for the first time was shocking. I didn't know who I was referring to. I thought, I don't want to say that – it makes it real.

It is this combination of factors that in my experience has caused many to press a 'pause' button on life; to put major decisions and commitments on hold as they wait for a child to stop the pain. The sadness, anxiety and lack of contentment can mass together to create a downward spiral of unproductive grief.

Battling with God

Hope

The diagnosis that I had serious subfertility issues because of low ovarian reserve rocked my world as nothing has before or since. I am angry with God; it has really affected our relationship and I hope others can pray me home again.

As people like Hope express, one of the hardest things about trying to accept infertility as the years go on is that it can feel like you're giving up. But if we dig a bit further, our thinking may go something like this: If I'm honest, I don't want God's will to be done through my childlessness. I want God's will to be done by me having a child.

There's a battle here. It's a battle between wanting what I want and wanting what God wants. I wonder if this is what submission to God at this point looks like. It is about giving up, but it's about giving up the control over wanting what I want. It's about giving up the desire to decide what's in God's interests. It's praying to be used by him, with or without a child or family, to help achieve his purposes for me and for the church.

As I (Sue) struggled to deal with some of these challenges, I read a book by Lois Flowers which really identified the questions I needed to ask myself. These were: would you be ready to pray for God to take away your desire for a child and family, or lessen it, in order to cope with this stage in life? Would you be willing to pray for God's will to be done through your infertility?[1]

This was a turning point for me. But it's important that you don't feel a load of guilt if you just can't pray this at the moment. There's a step before this that might help if you can't honestly pray this now, something along the lines of: 'Lord, praying for you to take away my desire for a child is just too painful, so help me to get to the point where I can pray this. Give me renewed trust in your goodness and strengthen my faith in you honestly to submit these desires to your good will, so that your purposes can be worked out.'

Tim
Over the years we have wrestled with faith in God in the face of ongoing infertility. IVF treatments have not resulted in a sustained pregnancy and live birth. This has led to frustration when seeing God answer the prayers of others.

As people like Tim show, getting to this part of the story can be exhausting. Fighting with oneself, struggling with conflicting emotions and coping with real grief is wearisome. It still feels a very lonely struggle, and may feel as though God has forgotten you as time goes on. Take to heart God's response to Jacob and Israel's complaint and accusation to God that their way was hidden, their cause unnoticed by God.

> Why do you say, O Jacob,
>   and complain, O Israel,
> 'My way is hidden from the LORD;
>   my cause is disregarded by my God'?
> Do you not know?
>   Have you not heard?
> The LORD is the everlasting God,
>   the Creator of the ends of the earth.
> He will not grow tired or weary,
>   and his understanding no-one can fathom.
> He gives strength to the weary
>   and increases the power of the weak.
> Even youths grow tired and weary,
>   and young men stumble and fall;
> but those who hope in the LORD
>   will renew their strength.
> They will soar on wings like eagles;
>   they will run and not grow weary,
>   they will walk and not be faint.
> (Isaiah 40:27–31)

God is able to give strength to the weary. It's a strength that is given to us as we hope in the Lord during testing times. It's strength to help us endure this trial.

We may doubt God's purposes. We may find it difficult to understand how anything could be more important or more significant than having a baby. Yet God's purposes for us are actually the same as his purposes were for Abraham during uncertain times – Abraham, who was 'strengthened in his faith and gave glory to God' (Romans 4:20). Above all else, these are the two most valuable things that God wants for us. He wants our faith to be strengthened and for us to give him glory, throughout the trials we face. So be assured that God will not grow tired of your struggles, but is there to strengthen the weary.

How do I let go of my dreams?

Kath

We have been very open with my parents and in-laws and they have all been very understanding. But it is them that I weep for most, I think. I somehow think that I am letting them down. I know they desire to have grandchildren and I want them to have grandchildren. I long for the day when they can bounce their grandchildren on their knees, when they can take the grandchildren on holiday or have the joy of seeing them pass exams. I feel guilty that I am not able to produce children for them to enjoy.

Trudy

Christmas is not easy, and the evenings, when I imagine bathing my children and putting them to bed, are hard too.

Part of the chronic grief of childlessness is dealing with the dreams that you have had for a family of your own: dreams that involved a future house, meal times, holidays, school runs; dreams that of themselves are not at all wrong. But these dreams are now threatened by infertility.

A kind of paradox can happen, that as each month or year goes by, the more unlikely it seems that you will attain your dream, the stronger this dream becomes. The danger here is not so much the dream itself, but how much you want it. What was once a hope and a longing becomes something you can't live without. This dream motivates you; it gives you a reason to get up in the morning. You become totally preoccupied by it and it starts to make demands of you – such as following all kinds of leads to increase your chances of conceiving: this may be diet related, vitamin supplements, exercise regimes, regimenting your sex life. Some of these may start off as useful things which may be sensible to pursue, but they can so easily become something you begin to obsess about or have rigidly to control. This dream has taken you over. There is a growing desperation, where all desire is focused on this one goal.

Paul David Tripp puts it like this: 'Your pursuit of the dream gives you meaning and purpose. The accomplishment of the dream gives you identity. You will even judge God's faithfulness by whether or not he gives you the dream.'² If you recognize this snowball effect, then you need to ask, 'What has actually captured my heart here? What is it that I really want out of life?' One way of trying to identify this is to complete the following sentence: 'If only I had . . . then I would be happy.' As Tripp goes on, 'Your dream has begun to compete with the rulership of your heart.' So it may be worth asking . . .

Who rules my heart?

It's worth being brutally honest with yourself. What is at stake is a question about who rules your heart. This dream could compete with God for the rule of your heart, because if you believe that if only you had a family then you would be happy, it will legitimize all sorts of behaviour in the pursuit of that aim.

Although the desire for a family is itself not wrong, getting to the point where you believe you will not be happy or fulfilled until this happens means that a radical displacement has occurred in your heart.

This is what the Bible calls idolatry – when we desire something else other than the worship of God first and foremost. Julian Hardyman's book, *Idols: God's Battle for Our Hearts*, reveals the origin and extent of our idol worship:

> At the root of all our life choices is a false belief system centred on an idol (or three) – the false belief that something other than God can give us the life, the joy, the hope and the truth that only God can give. The Bible calls this a lie . . . we believe the lie and dig the cistern and drink the water.[3]

Idols in this day and age are not generally made of wood as they were in the time of the Old Testament. Then, idols functioned to take Israel's eye and heart off serving God first. They provided an alternative for worship, with disastrous effects. The effects were to make the Israelites like the idol: blind, deaf and dumb. The effects of allowing this happiness idol to rule our hearts today will also be disastrous. Desiring that happiness idol is not a neutral desire. It will not leave you unscathed. It will take over your heart if you let it. 'Idols do not improve us, they reduce us, they hollow us out. They leave us less than we were. Less human, less satisfied, less of what we could be and should be. And they do this by making us like themselves.'[4]

The dream's promise of providing complete happiness and fulfilment in a family is empty and elusive. We are chasing a dream that looks like the real thing we were made for but is actually counterfeit. We were made for relationship, a close family-type relationship where we know and are known intimately. It is right to desire this closeness, but we need to recognize that having our dream family will never meet this need. We will be ever trying to grasp something unattainable. Our deep need for relationship can come only from knowing God through Christ his Son, partially now, and fully in eternity. We don't really believe God when he says that all we need to do is love him with all our heart, soul, mind and strength. Admitting this is the first step in denying this idol, this dream of future happiness and its power.

Guard your heart against bitterness

Sam and Polly

When people ask how many children we have, of course we say, 'Two', but often we want to say, 'Three'. Depending on the situation, we do sometimes say that our third was stillborn. She has been part of our family and we occasionally think about how old she would have been and what she might have been doing. We nevertheless do not allow these passing thoughts, quite legitimate in themselves, to degenerate into sinful self-indulgence.

Sam and Polly show how easy it could be for justifiable responses, in their case grief, to cause us to turn away from God. Having a deep but unrealized desire for a child can lead to bitterness and hardness. According to Hebrews 3:12, bitterness or hardness come from having 'a sinful, unbelieving heart that turns away from the living God'. It's a slippery slope where the natural desire for children may change over time into something that brings about hardness of heart, causing us to turn away from the living God.

It can be easy to feel God is withholding something good and natural, and we can easily cool off towards him. We feel let down by God. We stop trusting in his promise that 'in all things God works for the good of those who love him, who have been called according to his purpose' (Romans 8:28). This coolness and disappointment deceive us into turning away from God, leading to a hardening of our hearts.

Ultimately I think this comes down to whom I continue to place my trust in. I can continue to trust in God and his promises during testing times, or I can place my trust in what is tangible around me, be that the prospect of a child, or a spouse, or my own personality, coping skills, independence or circumstances. Trusting God is acknowledging daily that he is for us (Romans 8:31) in all of life's circumstances. My circumstances have been ordered to bring about my good, to be conformed to the likeness of Christ (verse 29). His ways are for my best, even in this testing time. Being infertile now is not plan B. It's not second best.

The Bible is full of warnings, in both the Old Testament and the New, to guard our hearts. Through these warnings, I (Sue) realized that I had to acknowledge my lack of trust in God when I saw my dream for a family was not going to be delivered. It was then that I saw that I needed to let go of this dream of 'happiness' as defined by having children, and try to pray that God would show me how else I can serve him. Yes, children will undoubtedly bring great joy and huge fulfilment. But the joy is a God-given by-product, and not something in and of itself to be chased after at all costs and to all ends.

Acknowledging that God alone sees the whole picture and knows our future frees us from the tyranny of being in charge. God alone is. Believing in God's promises during this time of testing, and encouraging others to do so, helps insure us against hardened hearts. He alone is faithful and true to his promises.

It is only in becoming more like Christ and trusting in his promises that we will have a glimpse of the true contentment that is ours to come when we are fully reunited with Christ.

God has not short-changed you by not giving you children. He is fundamentally in charge of every single event in your life, capable of bringing about what he considers best for you, for the sake of his glory. This means that your position now is not a 'mistake'. You can't get away with saying, 'Well, I feel I could really serve God better as a mother.' In effect what you are saying is that God has made a mistake, and the fact that you don't have the child or family you long for means that you are not able to give him your full service. Graham Beynon puts it like this: 'Beginning with me and my needs and then asking God to fill them keeps me at the centre. It makes Jesus revolve around me and what I want. Instead I have to allow Jesus to redefine me totally and tell me what my needs really are.'[5]

God looks at the heart

In all life events it's my response to God that's important, because life events can cause me to thank God for his kindness or they can be a source of grumbling. See how Proverbs 30:7–9 describes this tension where wealth and poverty are concerned:

> Two things I ask of you, O LORD;
>> do not refuse me before I die:
> Keep falsehood and lies far from me;
>> give me neither poverty nor riches,
>> but give me only my daily bread.
> Otherwise, I may have too much and disown you
>> and say, 'Who is the LORD ?'
> Or I may become poor and steal,
>> and so dishonour the name of my God.

Just as both wealth and poverty may lead to a poor response to God because our hearts are prone to being unthankful, so it is with children or childlessness. Both those with and without children have the same responsibility. It's a responsibility to relinquish any self-determined control over what we think would define our individual happiness. God looks at our hearts, whatever our circumstances. Mary's response captures this struggle to examine her heart:

Mary

We are members of a wonderful church family and have great positive relationships with a number of children. I think my focus is beginning to become more outward looking and Christ-focused again rather than self-focused. But we are at the very beginning of learning to accept that our lives won't necessarily be shaped by having a family and all the milestones that this brings, so we will therefore be praying and seeking guidance for a different journey and opportunities.

We may not have full understanding now of all of God's ways, but the Old Testament prophet Habakkuk reminds us of what to do as we wait for God's full salvation and a fully restored relationship with him: 'The righteous will live by his faith' (2:4b). Habakkuk finishes his prophecy by describing what this looks like when we face barren fields and hunger:

> Though the fig-tree does not bud
>> and there are no grapes on the vines,
> though the olive crop fails
>> and the fields produce no food,
> though there are no sheep in the pen
>> and no cattle in the stalls,

yet I will rejoice in the LORD,
    I will be joyful in God my Saviour.

The Sovereign LORD is my strength;
    he makes my feet like the feet of a deer,
    he enables me to go on the heights.
(Habakkuk 3:17–19)

It's a tough challenge to be called to rejoice in the Lord during these times, but God in his sovereignty makes it possible for us to go on as we rejoice. He alone is our strength.

15 Hope for the future?

Trudy

I have to stop worrying about the future, being widowed and alone with no children to comfort me.

Trudy's struggle shows that the pain of infertility is often projected into the future. I (Sue) echoed this. I came to dread the next twenty years. Facing a future without children brought fresh anxieties about who would look after me in my old age. This is also the case for parents of children who are trying to conceive.

Carol

The anguish of being of grandmotherly age without grandchildren, when others have nine or ten – I know someone with eighteen – is anguish, no more, no less. To pretend otherwise is dishonesty. You look at other grandmothers – you think you are as 'good' as they are, and God blesses them but he doesn't bless you. I am happy to say that what Elkanah said to Hannah was echoed by my husband. His attitude was, 'Am I not more to you than ten grandsons?' But how I longed for one grandson.

Those such as Carol face the deep disappointment of not having grandchildren, and all that they were looking forward to in their later years. Theirs is a double pain: coping with their son or daughter's infertility and also coming to terms with their own sense of loss at not being grandparents. Peer pressure may come into it too. Parents of married couples face questions about when their son or daughter is going to start a family. They see others' joy at becoming grandparents with its incumbent roles and responsibilities. They grieve, but often can't express it.

The Christian's hope at this stage, when it all seems a bit final, is that there is something better than having children now.

Better than sons and daughters

In the Old Testament, a eunuch was an officer in the court or household of a ruler. He was generally assigned to the women's quarters and was often emasculated. Eunuchs, denied the ability to father children, were told in Isaiah 56:3 not to complain, 'I am only a dry tree.'

For this is what the LORD says:

'To the eunuchs who keep my Sabbaths,
   who choose what pleases me
   and hold fast to my covenant –
to them I will give within my temple and its walls
   a memorial and a name
   better than sons and daughters;
I will give them an everlasting name
   that will not be cut off.'
(Isaiah 56:4–5)

God graciously promised a salvation which was an everlasting name, better than sons or daughters. In Revelation 14:1 we find out what this name will be. For the people of God, his servants, '[the Lamb's] name and his Father's name' will be 'on their foreheads'. This is about our identity and reputation being bound up utterly with who God is. We will be truly his, for ever. We need to grasp the wonder and majesty of this everlasting identity to give us hope as we wait in this world now.

One of my (Sue's) fears is that when I die I will soon be forgotten, as I have no offspring to remember me. The prospect of the family name ceasing can cause sadness and anxiety. But great comfort can be drawn from our knowledge of God.

Your past, present and future in God's hands

Anxiety can be crippling. Anxiety about the future can make you freeze in the present. At its heart, anxiety is really about control. David Powlison devotes a chapter to the subject of anxiety in his book *Seeing with New Eyes* which covers the topic far more fully than can be done here. He writes, 'all the things we worry about are what we want but could lose'. He goes on, 'The illusion of control lurks inside your anxiety. Anxiety and control are two sides of the same coin. When we can't control something, we worry about it.'[1]

David Powlinson helpfully looks at Luke 12:22–34 in detail and in particular draws out the amazing promise of provision in verse 32 for those who worry or are anxious. 'Do not be afraid, little flock, for your Father has been pleased to give you the kingdom.' He writes, 'It's the only place in the Bible where that phrase, "little flock", is used. It's a vivid picture of a flock of sheep small enough that the shepherd knows all their names, their personalities, and what each one faces.'

This is our certain hope – that God knows us intimately and he knows what we need. In Deuteronomy 31 the people of Israel were given the news that their leader Moses was no longer going to lead them. Faced with the uncertainty, fear and terror of impending attack from their enemies, Moses said in verse 6, 'Be strong and courageous. Do not be afraid or terrified because of them, for the LORD your God goes with you; he will never leave you nor forsake you.' This promise was used by the writer of Hebrews to reiterate God's faithful promise to be with us always, when we are tempted to think we don't have what we need in life. The apostle Paul's confidence in 2 Timothy 4:18 was in the Lord who 'will bring me safely to his heavenly kingdom'. This time on earth is short. Our days of struggle, anxiety and temptation to give up will end. God holds your past, present and future in his hands.

So as we look ahead to a future which is uncertain, do not be anxious. Hold on to God's promises not to leave or forget us. Remember Psalm 9:10: 'Those who know your name will trust in you, for you, LORD, have never forsaken those who seek you.' When you have died you may not have children to remember you, but God has promised never to forget you. Your life with him is everlasting.

Opportunities

Accepting your infertility may take time, but with God's grace it can be done. At times it may feel that you have only a very tenuous grasp of this acceptance. It is hard to look back over life and accept that this is not where you wanted to be, and it's hard to put to death your dreams.

Some of our friends have regretted how much time and energy they have spent on trying to have children. Unfocused regret can freeze you in the present, rendering you unable to forgive yourself or look ahead. But, as Paul David Tripp writes, regret may be a tool by which God administers grace: 'Because grace calls you to see, it will lead you to regret . . . It is a sweet grace to see, to regret and to run to the One who makes all things new.'[2]

It is no accident that you are where you are now. God in his sovereignty has ordained this path. You now face a different future from what you had hoped for. Accept that what God has brought to an end may bring sadness, but this is a necessary step towards a new beginning. God is a God of restoration, of new beginnings, of new life. It might be that this is the time you need to ask God to show you how else you can serve him, what areas of service you could develop that you may not have thought of before. And as you continue on in Christian ministry, you will do so having been refined and trained by God as you have struggled with infertility. With God's help, you have more to offer the church now than you had before.

Over time, some couples have been able to take on new responsibilities that would not have otherwise been possible had they had children. Here are just two examples.

Trudy

The Lord has been very good to us . . . There have been unexpected joys too: I have great pleasure in being involved with a family from Bangladesh who live nearby. I'll never forget the day, seven years ago, when I met them. Several small heads appeared one by one around the door. I felt like Maria in The Sound of Music *as each child was presented to me. What started off as me being a homework helper for the five children has developed into a lasting friendship, particularly with the two teenage girls. I love them dearly, and by happy coincidence, the feeling appears to be mutual. I call them my part-time daughters.*

Tom

Some close friends asked if they could nominate us to become the guardians of their children in the event of their deaths. That was an enormous privilege . . . Not having children has enabled us to get involved in things at church which might otherwise have proved impractical.

Taking on new responsibilities that would not have been possible with children is not second best. These are new opportunities to serve which God in his sovereignty has ordained for you to do.

Reflecting on chapters 14 – 15

Something to read

Read Hebrews 12 and 13. How does the writer of Hebrews help us guard against weariness as we continue to persevere as Christians?

Something to do

Have a go at filling in the sentence, 'If only I had . . . . then I would be happy.'

A conversation to have

Talk to a good friend about how you could use your skills and gifts to serve the church as you are now.

For friends and pastors

Build up relationships of trust and acceptance, because if you are going to minister to someone with infertility, you are in it for the long haul.

Ask specifically how you can pray.

For further reading

Paul David Tripp, *Lost in the Middle: Midlife and the Grace of God* (Shepherd Press, 2004).
Julian Hardyman, *Idols: God's Battle for Our Hearts* (Inter-Varsity Press, 2010).

Conclusion

What should I expect from now on?

Trudy

Infertility is a journey – often a painful one, but it does get easier. God in his grace can use this disappointment to bless us and make us more like him. I don't have answers to the question 'Why me, Lord?', but I do trust his character, and believe that he is good and faithful, and I know that still believing this, despite my sadness, is somehow precious in his sight. Not being a mother will always be a sadness to me, but it does get a little easier, and I do enjoy the life I have. I don't know why God said 'no' to us, but I do trust his love for me.

Helen has faced multiple miscarriages. This is an extract from her diary:

On Sunday we were on welcoming and crèche duty at church. I found that day really difficult as we were very tired, but also because everyone is pregnant or has just had babies. I am happy for my friends, but at the same time I am sad that I am not pregnant. I am starting to become obsessed with it again. I thought I was pregnant last week before my period came, but I'm not, and I am now on the last days of a very heavy period . . . I am thinking about getting pregnant all day every day. It is getting me down and I keep bursting into tears. I cannot control the tears. I am not sure what is going on. Could it be period hormones? I don't know. But whatever it is, I'm feeling sad. Really sad in fact. People have noticed that I'm not my 'bubbly self'.

In thinking about what might happen to that desire for children and what we can expect in this life, women like Trudy, and men have said that they have come to a place of acceptance, some after many years. In my (Sue's) experience, the rawness has decreased over time. But clearly for Helen the rawness is still palpable. It will be different for each one of us. For many the fight continues. We will struggle afresh with feelings we thought we had put to bed: sadness, temptation to anger, jealousy, envy. We'll encounter some who have experienced infertility go on to have the children and families they longed for. Effortless fertility in others which produces a bounty of beautiful babies will mock us and tempt us to question God's love for us over and over again.

This is not to sound discouraging, but instead realistic. There may not be a 'neat' conclusion to our grief. There's a tension in Trudy's trust in God's love, as it is coupled with recurrent sadness at not being a mother. We may not experience the closure we long for. We may never be given a full understanding of why this has happened, and so for many of us, the pain will remain in some form.

But one day we will have all the answers when we know God fully. Our role now is to keep trusting in our heavenly Father for all things. Mary's experience speaks of God's constant love for her.

Mary
I have felt my faith has definitely fluctuated but have never doubted that our God is one of love, compassion, grace and mercy,

although for some reason, whether that be due to the world and humankind's failings, we do not always receive the healing we think we need.

In order to help us live now amid the sadness of infertility, we can take heart from Paul, who writes in Ephesians 1:13–14 that we have 'a seal, the promised Holy Spirit, who is a deposit guaranteeing our inheritance [of these blessings] until the redemption of those who are God's possession'. God's blessing is to keep us going as Christians, fixed on the hope and looking forward to all that is to come, and not giving up on him. Paul tells us in 2 Corinthians 4:7–9 that as our endurance will be tested, we will feel it is very fragile. But God is faithful.

But we have this treasure in jars of clay to show that this all-surpassing power is from God and not from us. We are hard pressed on every side, but not crushed; perplexed, but not in despair; persecuted, but not abandoned; struck down, but not destroyed.

Kate

I have to admit that the years of infertility were among the most spiritually satisfying of my life. Through all the disappointment, I always felt the Lord was there, and his love seemed to transcend the pain. On one occasion, during an IVF cycle, I was sitting in the kitchen talking to a young member of our church group, explaining about Christianity. I realized that all was not well and excused myself to go to the bathroom, only to discover that the cycle had failed. On returning I continued the discussion, and this young person subsequently became a Christian. It felt to me that as a potential life was lost, so another had been born into the kingdom of God. What grace, what love!

Kate's story is a great example of a faith and a joy that do not waver in the face of terrible disappointment: a faith that triumphs in God's work of a new birth, even when it is not the birth of the child that she greatly desires.

God is working for our good. Often it will not feel like that. Our experience deceives us if we listen to it alone. God's Word is absolutely clear that God is for us; he has ordained everything for our good. As you pray, hold out this verse to him, trusting that he will do this. 'And we know that in all things God works for the good of those who love him, who have been called according to his purpose' (Romans 8:28).

Bibliography

Christopher Ash, *Married for God: Making Your Marriage the Best It Can Be* (Inter-Varsity Press, 2007).

Stephen C. Barton, 'Living as Families in the Light of the New Testament', *Interpretation* 52/2, 1998, p. 138.

Graham Beynon, *Mirror, Mirror: Discover Your True Identity in Christ* (Inter-Varsity Press, 2008).

Daniel I. Block. 'Marriage and Family in Ancient Israel' in Ken Campbell (ed.), *Marriage and Family in the Biblical World* (Inter-Varsity Press, 2004), p. 38.

Guy Brandon, *Just Sex: Is It Ever Just Sex?* (Inter-Varsity Press, 2009).

J. D. Douglas (ed.), *Illustrated Bible Dictionary* (Inter-Varsity Press, 1987).

Michael R. Emlet, 'When It Won't Go Away: A Biblical Response to Chronic Pain', *Journal of Biblical Counseling*, Winter 2005.

Lois Flowers, *Infertility: Finding God's Peace in the Journey* (Harvest House, 2003).

John Gray, *Men Are From Mars, Women Are From Venus: A Practical Guide to Improving Communication and Getting What You Want in Your Relationships* (Thorsons, 1993).

Julian Hardyman, *Idols: God's Battle for Our Hearts* (Inter-Varsity Press, 2010).

Kimberly and Philip Monroe, 'The Bible and the Pain of Infertility', *Journal of Biblical Counseling*, Winter 2005; 50–58.

NIV Thematic Study Bible (Hodder and Stoughton, 1996).

John Piper and Justin Taylor, *Suffering and the Sovereignty of God* (Crossway, 2006).

David Powlison, *Seeing with New Eyes: Counseling and the Human Condition Through the Lens of Scripture* (P & R Publishing, 2003).

Andrew Reid, *Salvation Begins: Reading Genesis Today* (Aquila Press, 2000).

J. B. Stanford et al., *Journal of the American Board of Family Medicine* (2008), 21:375–384.

Paul David Tripp, *Lost in the Middle: Midlife and the Grace of God* (Shepherd Press, 2004).

Lauren Winner, *Real Sex: The Naked Truth about Chastity* (Brazos Press, 2005).

www.cmf.org.uk: follow link to 'Early life' and then 'Reproductive technologies' to find several recent publications and articles from the Christian Medical Fellowship.

John Wyatt, *Matters of Life and Death: Human Dilemmas in the Light of the Christian Faith* (Inter-Varsity Press, 2009).

Robert Young, *Young's Analytical Concordance to the Bible* (Hendrickson, 2002; originally published 1879).

Further reading and resources

Kirsten Birkett, *The Essence of Family* (Matthias Media, 2004).

D. A. Carson, *How Long, O Lord? Reflections on Suffering and Evil* (Inter-Varsity Press, 1990).

Rosemary and Barry Jubraj, *Infertility: The Silent and Unseen Issue* (RoperPenberthy Publishing, 2007).

Graham McFarlane and Pete Moore, 'What is a person?', Christian Medical Fellowship files, Number 10 (2000).

John Piper and Justin Taylor, *Suffering and the Sovereignty of God* (Crossway, 2006).

Lesley Regan, *Miscarriage: What Every Woman Needs to Know* (Orion, 2001).

Jennifer Saake, *Hannah's Hope: Seeking God's Heart in the Midst of Infertility, Miscarriage, and Adoption Loss* (NavPress, 2005).

Al Stewart, *Men: Firing Through All of Life* (Blue Bottle Books, 2007).

Information on adoption in the UK and international adoption from the UK: www.direct.gov.uk and search using 'adoption' or type in www.direct.gov.uk/en/Parents/Adoptionfosteringandchildrenincare and follow 'adoption' link followed by 'intercountry adoption' to find legal and statutory requirements for adopting overseas. www.bemyparent.org.uk is the link to the newspaper carrying profiles of children available for adoption in the UK (be aware that these children are often those who are harder to place).

Fertility guidance: www.nice.org.uk/guidance

Natural fertility information: www.naprotechnology.co.uk

Notes

1. Introduction

1 NICE (National Institute of Clinical Excellence) fertility guidance: www.nice.org.uk/guidance

2 C. L. R. Barratt and I. D. Cooke (eds.), *Donor Insemination* (Cambridge University Press, 1993), p. 13, citing Connolly, Edelmann and Cooke, 1987.

Section 1: Where is God in all this pain?

2. Why me?

1 Andrew Reid, *Salvation Begins: Reading Genesis Today* (Aquila Press, 2000), p. 29.

2 Andrew Reid, *Salvation Begins: Reading Genesis Today* (Aquila Press, 2000), p. 34.

5. This hurts

1 Paul David Tripp, *Lost in the Middle: Midlife and the Grace of God* (Shepherd Press, 2004), p. 151.

2 A. D. Domar, P. C. Zuttermeister and R. Friedman, 'The Psychological Impact of Infertility: A Comparison with Patients with Other Medical Conditions', *Journal of Psychosomatic Obstetrics & Gynecology* 14 (1993) Suppl: 45–52: PMID 8142988.

Section 2: Coping with the stress of childlessness

6. Who am I, without a family?

1 Daniel I. Block, 'Marriage and Family in Ancient Israel' in Ken Campbell (ed.), *Marriage and Family in the Biblical World* (Inter-Varsity Press, 2004), p. 38.

2 Kimberly and Philip Monroe, 'The Bible and the Pain of Infertility', *Journal of Biblical Counseling*, Winter 2005, pp. 50–58.

8. Keeping marriage strong

1 Christopher Ash, *Married for God: Making Your Marriage the Best It Can Be* (Inter-Varsity Press, 2007), p. 15.

2 Church of England Alternative Service Book (ASB), 1980.

3 Guy Brandon, *Just Sex: Is It Ever Just Sex?* (Inter-Varsity Press, 2009), p. 98.

4 Lauren Winner, *Real Sex* (Brazos Press, 2005), p. 80.

5 Christopher Ash, *Married for God* (Inter-Varsity Press, 2007), p. 77.

9. Real men experience infertility

1 John Gray, *Men Are From Mars, Women Are From Venus: A Practical Guide to Improving Communication and Getting What You Want in Your Relationships* (Thorsons, 1993).

10. Grieving miscarriage, late-term pregnancy loss and secondary infertility

1 New Living Translation.

2 There is a helpful chapter by Dustin Shramek in John Piper and Justin Taylor's book, *Suffering and the Sovereignty of God*, entitled 'Waiting for the morning during the long night of weeping' which considers this in more detail (Crossway, 2006).

3 Kimberly and Philip Monroe, 'The Bible and the Pain of
   Infertility', *Journal of Biblical Counseling*, Winter 2005,
   pp. 50–58.

Section 3: How can the professionals help?

1 John Wyatt, *Matters of Life and Death: Human Dilemmas in
   the Light of the Christian Faith* (Inter-Varsity Press, 2009),
   p. 86.

12. Treatment

1 John Wyatt, *Matters of Life and Death: Human Dilemmas in
   the Light of the Christian Faith* (Inter-Varsity Press, 2009),
   p. 106.
2 Christian Medical Fellowship website: www.cmf.org.uk
   Enter 'reproductive technologies' into search box at the top of
   the home page to find recent articles by the CMF on topics such
   as egg freezing, donor gametes and the ethics of assisted
   conception.

Section 4: The long unknown

14. Is acceptance possible?

1 Lois Flowers, *Infertility: Finding God's Peace in the Journey*
   (Harvest House, 2003), pp. 66–67.
2 Paul David Tripp, *Lost in the Middle: Midlife and the Grace of God*
   (Shepherd Press, 2004), p. 145.
3 Julian Hardyman, *Idols: God's Battle for Our Hearts* (Inter-Varsity
   Press, 2010), p. 169.
4 Julian Hardyman, *Idols: God's Battle for Our Hearts* (Inter-Varsity
   Press, 2010), p. 141.
5 Graham Beynon, *Mirror, Mirror: Discover Your True Identity in
   Christ* (Inter-Varsity Press, 2008). p. 121.

15. Hope for the future?

1 David Powlison, *Seeing with New Eyes: Counseling and the Human Condition Through the Lens of Scripture* (P & R Publishing, 2003), p. 115.
2 Paul David Tripp, *Lost in the Middle: Midlife and the Grace of God* (Shepherd Press, 2004), pp. 338–339.